Eat Local for Less

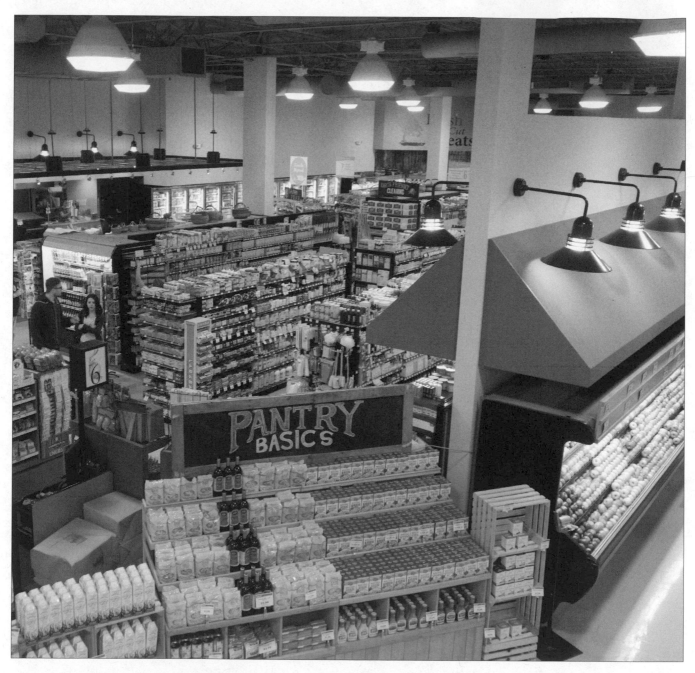

Abundant local goods are sold at the Common Market in Frederick, Md. (see page 117).

Eat Local for Less

The Ultimate Guide to Opting Out
of Our Broken Industrial Food System

Julie Castillo

Ruka Press®

Washington, DC

Disclaimer: The author and publisher do not assume responsibility for the outcome of any course of action suggested in this book. Visiting farms, businesses, or websites; trying foods, alcoholic beverages, or recipes; cooking, gardening, animal husbandry, beekeeping, volunteering, or any other activities suggested or recommended herein, including those suggested for children, are to be undertaken solely at the reader's discretion and risk. Check with a physician before starting any exercise regimens, dietary changes, or activities that may place your health at risk.

A Note About Names: In order to protect their privacy, I've changed the names of some of the individuals mentioned in this book. I've used my own name, though, in order to show that I fully stand behind the words I've written. The names of all farmers, business owners, authors, scientists, and experts who are mentioned in this book also remain unchanged.

Photo credits: Title page: Jeff Stevens; page 8: Tory Cowles; page 148: Steve Bill; page 208: Steve Alswang; page 254: Kristi Janzen; page 270: Tony Brusco.

Library of Congress Cataloging-in-Publication Data
Castillo, Julie, 1965–
    Eat local for less : the ultimate guide to opting out of our broken industrial food system / Julie Castillo.
        pages cm
    Includes index.
    ISBN 978-0-9855748-6-4 (pbk. : alk. paper)—ISBN (invalid) 978-0-9855748-7-1 (pdf)
—ISBN 978-0-9855748-8-8 (epub)—ISBN (invalid) 978-0-9855748-9-5 (kindle)
 1. Cooking (Natural foods) 2. Local foods. 3. Nutrition. 4. Health. I. Title.
    TX741.C374 2015
    641.3'02—dc23

                                           2014044943

First edition published 2015 by Ruka Press,® PO Box 1409, Washington, DC 20013.
www.rukapress.com

10 9 8 7 6 5 4 3 2 1

Printed in the United States of America

Design by Sensical Design & Communication

Table of Contents

Index of Recipes

This book is dedicated to the three people who sit at my dinner table every night, who are the source of my happiness every day: My husband, Al, and my sons, Benjamin and Phillip. It's also dedicated to Bonnie, Kristi, Kathy, and Laura, and to the memory of sweet Felicia. How lucky I was to have walked into the Writing Center that day.

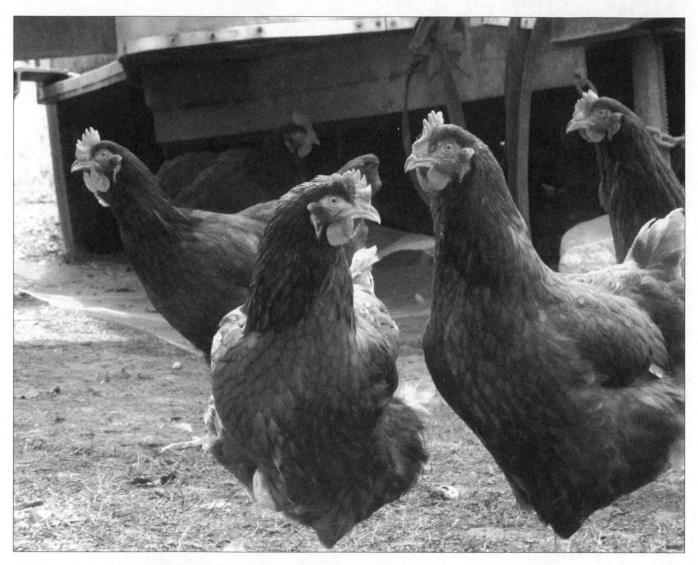

Pastured hens strut at Miolea Farm in Adamstown, Md.

Eat Local for Less

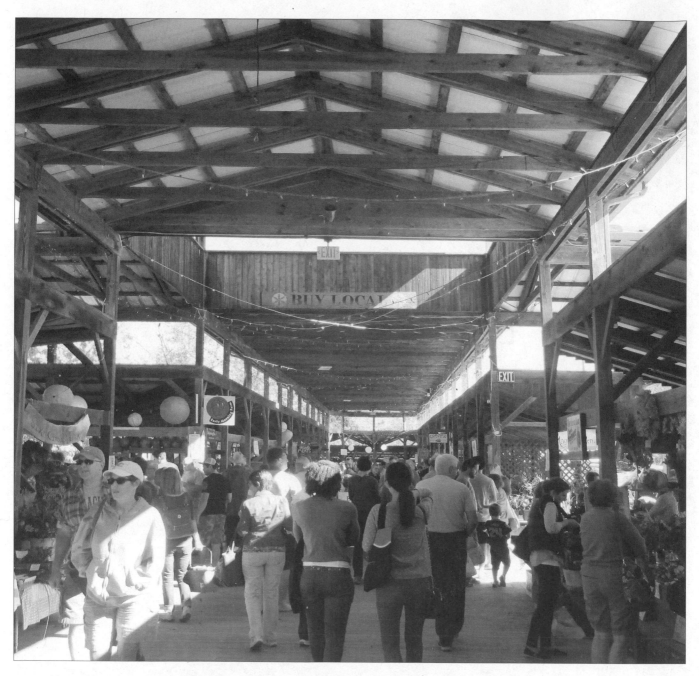

The Ithaca Farmers Market in Ithaca, N.Y. has been a local food destination since 1973.

First Thoughts

Thinking of Opting Out?

Tell me what you eat, and I will tell you what you are. —*Jean Anthelme Brillat-Savarin*

"D o you eat?"

This was how my husband's Uncle Nick welcomed me into his house the first time I met him—his standard words of salutation, I learned later, usually followed by, "Do you like meat? 'Cause that's all we got here."

His greeting was at once disarming and charming. It made for instant rapport with anyone who walked in his door because, well, who doesn't love to eat? Uncle Nick followed up the introductions by sitting me down to a heaping plate of homemade *tostones* and Puerto Rican style braised pork shoulder. Two minutes after I walked in the door, I was part of the family.

For humans, eating is not just a means to sustenance. It's also an expression of kinship. It connects us to each other: as Uncle Nick knows, we all eat, and we like to do it *together*. Anthropology, the scientific study of human beings, tells us that food is a key to understanding the structure of any society. How a group of people obtains its food influences everything from its art, music, gender roles, and family life to its political structure, economic system, and religion. Our foodways define who we are. For humans, and no other creature that we know of, it also carries meaning. What we eat, how we eat, and even *when* we eat make a statement about the worldview we share.

So here we are, more than 317 million twenty-first century Americans. What do our foodways say about us? According to a study published by the National Institutes of Health, we eat approximately five billion fast food hamburgers a year. Nearly every car sold in the United States today comes standard-equipped with several soft drink holders, and the national auto parts retailer Pep Boys will even sell you a french fry holder to go along with it. One in three American children is overweight. American adults eat approximately 150 pounds of sugar every year of their lives. According to the New York University Medical Center, family dinners have declined by 33 percent since the 1960s. Nearly half of us eat our meals alone. TV screens have become ubiquitous, not just in homes, but in many restaurants, blotting out with their incessant chatter all possibility of enjoying a quiet conversation with loved ones over dinner.

Do we like this picture of ourselves? Are the American foodways filling us with joy, bringing us closer together, bolstering our economic security, or providing us with robust health?

I'm guessing that this book caught your attention partly because the romance has gone out of your relationship with food. You probably have a childhood memory of biting into a ruby red tomato and having the taste explode on your tongue, yet the things they call by the same name in the grocery store today are insipid mush. You've thought, maybe it's because I'm getting old and my taste buds are dying. Maybe it's because the universe is in entropy and tomatoes have lost their tomato-ness. Or maybe, you've concluded, it's not your fault or the tomatoes' fault at all. Perhaps the blame lies with the massive corporations who grow tomatoes with the same conveyor-belt efficiency as the folks who manufacture tires or assemble microwave ovens.

It's probably not just the taste of your food that has you concerned. If you're like me, you get an ice-cold knot in your stomach when you read that, according to the Centers for Disease Control and Prevention, six hundred thousand Americans die from heart disease each year, or that 35.9 percent of American adults are obese. We are facing significant numbers of cases of high blood pressure, stroke, colorectal cancer, and diabetes. What's causing this? Could there be a connection between the state of our health and the food we're eating?

You're also probably aware that we've got even bigger problems looming: the way we're living is messing up our atmosphere, wrecking the fertility of our soil, and polluting our water and air. We are looking at a near future that could be dominated by climate change, rising energy costs, and shortages of everything from arable land to drinking water. Here, too, could these foreshadowed global crises have anything to do with the way we produce our food?

T here's more. You're probably aware that, in many places in today's world, people still go hungry. For them, there is no dollar menu to fall back on. Here in the United States, we produce about several hundred calories more per day *per person* than we could possibly stuff into ourselves. Yet, according to the Food and Agriculture Organization (FAO) of the United Nations, 870 million people across the globe don't get enough food each day to stay healthy. Approximately 220,000 per year die as a result. How is it that in 2015—in *the twenty-first century,* for God's sake—anyone can still starve to death? If we can allow this to happen, something is deeply out of whack about our global food priorities.

If you've followed this path of thinking, then your next step may have been to cast about for alternatives: if you don't want to eat highly processed shlock that undermines your health, pollutes the environment, depletes resources, and doesn't do a damn thing to address the root causes of hunger in the developing world, then what are your options?

That's when you might have discovered that there is this whole other food system that has been quietly producing delicious food in ways that not only don't wreck any ecosystems but actually *improve* some of them. These are the foods lovingly produced by small-scale farmers and family-run cottage businesses, not corporations. They're made in small quantities close to your community by people who cherish their land and work hard to keep it healthy.

The food these people produce don't add dioxin to your dinner; have seldom been linked to a major outbreak of E. coli; contain far less fat, cholesterol, salt, and sugar; and even give you more healthy omega-3 fatty acids. They don't depend on government subsidies, and they don't leverage small farmers in developing countries off their lands. They burn less fossil fuel in getting to you because they are grown within a hundred miles of your home. And when you sink your teeth into a tomato grown *this* way, you get the same juicy explosion of flavor you remember from childhood.

So you may have decided that this is the way you want to eat from now on. You're not alone. Many of us have come to the same conclusion in recent years—so many that we sometimes get called a movement.

But that's where you might have hit a snag. Let's say you've happened to score a head of organic, locally produced romaine lettuce in your local grocery store. You're happy—until you look at the price of the stuff. *Oy!* And of course, this just confirms what you've seen in the media, read on the Internet, and heard from friends: sure, local provender is a trendy treat for the foodie crowd, but *nobody can actually afford to eat this way*.

It's time to challenge that notion. If something is worth doing, there's got to be a way to do it. I've heard dozens of voices on TV, radio, Internet, and in print, grumbling that local and organic food was bound to be more expensive, and not one voice suggesting that *it could be cheaper*. I decided to be that one voice.

Sometimes people repeat a phrase so often that it comes to sound like the truth, and sooner or later, we may even accept it as such. And if we do, the brilliant start we Americans have made toward changing the way we obtain our food will never amount to more than a well-intentioned fad. We have an opportunity here, and I think we should run with it.

You don't need another book that tells you how to eat. *Eat Local for Less* isn't going to give you yet another set of rules about food choices. Instead, it will trust that you *have already made* that decision for yourself, and it will help you go about acting on that choice.

I want this book to empower you to rely on your own good sense and your storehouse of food knowledge. You may have come to believe that you don't have any such thing, but you have far more than you think. You've just let the media shake your confidence. If you relied on your own food wisdom, you wouldn't be as likely to eat their advertisers' overprocessed, nutritionally bankrupt products.

The impulse toward local food is part of a larger cultural shift. If the emphasis in our society in recent decades has been on commercialism and individual gain, then the pendulum appears poised to swing back toward community, family, and connections: shared household responsibilities, shared food-getting, shared cooking, and shared meals.

It's hard to equally serve both profits and relationships. For this reason, in many traditional cultures, money is treated with suspicion. It may be necessary to sustain life, but hold your nose and keep it at arm's length. Some cultures even practice rituals designed to keep the stress-causing effects of money at bay: anthropologist Janet Carsten says Malay fishermen give the money they make to their wives right away so that it can be absorbed into the household, where everything is shared. That way, it doesn't cause strife.

There's a level at which personal gain does seem to be at odds with interpersonal connections. According to the Bureau of Labor Statistics, the United

States' gross domestic product per capita rose from $17,747 in 1960 to $48,282 in 2011 (using 2011 U.S. dollars). Yet sociologist Robert Putnam, in his book *Bowling Alone*, argues that the number of beneficial connections we Americans have to other people has declined dramatically over the past two generations. Our "financial capital" has nearly tripled; our "social capital" has dropped.

Could it be that, while we've been busy chasing dollars, we've abdicated our bonds to each other?

I'm all for people making a healthy profit. There's nothing wrong with providing a great product or service and getting paid for it. But there is indeed something socially corrosive about maximizing profit at any cost, to the exclusion of all other goals.

I'm not trying to drag us back to a previous place in history, either. We can't return to an extinct model of society. We're not talking next-generation-June Cleavers. We need to invent a new kind of socioeconomic system that works with who we are becoming, and it needs to be one that places human needs and connections as the top priority, without exploiting, overburdening, or undervaluing any segment of our society.

One goal of this book is to open a dialogue about what comes next. We humans have, for the most part, plummeted headlong into our futures without deliberately constructing them. We've been like skydivers who jump from the plane without first ensuring that our parachutes were packed properly. That was fine when the metaphorical ground was far below, but now it's time to pull the ripcord. We've reached a point where there are so many of us, and where our technology is so pervasive, that we're doing things that could be catastrophic for our species and our planet.

President John F. Kennedy recognized this decades ago when, in his inaugural address, he claimed that humankind now possessed "the power to abolish all forms of human poverty and all forms of human life." In that case, we've reached an age where we have to be more careful. Maybe this is a good time to check our parachutes.

This book is not an indictment of what we're doing wrong; it's a celebration of the fact that we're starting to get it right. Its goal is to help as many people as possible act on the choices they've made to eat purposefully and buy responsibly.

In this book, I'm entertaining a new mind-set for the American foodways. I'm suggesting ways for us to grow, buy, cook, eat, and interact with food that are in harmony with who we truly intend to be. I'm proposing that our eating habits can be an expression of our respect for ourselves, our love for one another, and our awe of nature.

Here are the ultimate goals of our new foodways:

- Nutritious, safe, abundant, local, and accessible food for all people

- Food self-sufficiency for all communities

- Food that is grown sustainably and responsibly

- Multiple food streams and sources, to preserve true variety and choice

- Transparency of method: food growers who habitually show their farms and discuss their techniques with anyone who wants to know

- Food that is exchanged through responsible economics: in other words, a food economy that is need driven, rather than profit driven

- Agrarian wisdom, ecological knowledge, and cooking skills for all

We are the futuresmiths: by our eating habits we will forge the links of a new food chain. We are the bodhisattvas of the home-cooked meal: we hold open the kitchen door and invite everyone in to taste the simple goodness they've been missing. We do this, not because there are big bucks in it, but because it's what any thinking, feeling species does for its own, and for its planet, when it finally gets its act together.

Part 1

The Biggest Food Revolution Since the First Planted Seed

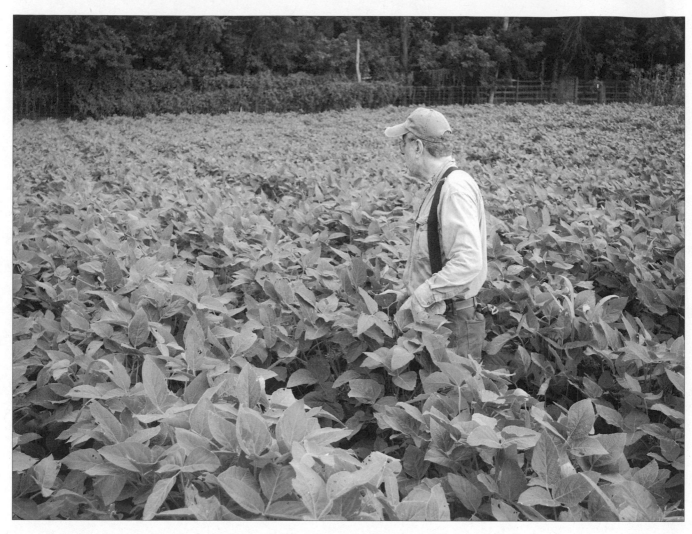

Rows of soybeans at Nick Maravell's Farm, Adamstown, Maryland.

1

A Suburban Family Goes Local

How We Broke Our Link in the Industrial Food Chain

'Tis not too late to seek a newer world. —*Alfred, Lord Tennyson*

When the universe hands you the same message from multiple directions, it's a good idea to pay attention.

I came to local food, not as a result of any single incident, but because a whole crowd of seemingly unrelated events pointed me this way. I first opened myself up to these experiences in 2012 when I officially declared myself a futurist. This struck me as the perfect year to embrace the future since, according to some interpretations of the Mayan calendar, we were about to run out of it.

Futurists hail from any number of scientific and creative disciplines, united by an interest in the challenges that lie ahead for humankind. I became a futurist because I wanted to make better use of my background in anthropology. My field suffers from a reputation for studying quaint, exotic, extinct, or nearly extinct cultures. People think we're obsessed with naked tribal folk dancing around with bones stuck through their noses. If you don't believe me, check out the picture on the cover of almost any anthropology textbook. To many people, "anthropology" is synonymous with "irrelevancy." Once, when I told a family friend I was studying anthropology, he replied, "Oh, you're going to dig up dead people?"

Anthropology is the study of *all* human beings, not just dead ones. Its prime directive, cultural relativism, states that you can't possibly understand any aspect of someone else's way of life if you judge it by the standards of your own. It doesn't rank one form of society as superior to another. Instead, it sees all societies as responses to environmental realities, and from that

Cultural Relativism

The anthropological assertion that it's impossible to understand someone else's way of life if you judge it by the standards of your own.

The Globalization of Agriculture

Just a few decades ago, nearly everyone ate seasonally: asparagus in springtime, tomatoes at midsummer, and apples in the fall. Today, most of what we Americans eat is available year-round, thanks to a global food system. It's convenient, but it comes to us at a high cost.

Much of what the average American eats today comes from large-scale farms thousands of miles away. Our reliance on imported and shipped foods marches in lockstep with our dependence on fossil fuels. And because importing food to wealthy countries is big business, it shifts small-scale landowners off of their land and relegates them to the role of low-paid laborer.

perspective, it offers a view of humankind you can't get anywhere else.

I started by framing a few questions: What are the biggest challenges facing humankind in the future? What human needs are going unmet?

As it turned out, the answers to these questions changed my life.

Becoming a futurist has meant coming face to face with many of my own misconceptions. I'd taken it as a given that Earth simply isn't able to feed all seven billion of us abundantly—why else would people be starving? I believed that only through large-scale industrial agriculture could food be made affordable. I didn't question the assumption that profit was the ultimate motivator in any large-scale economic system. It seemed obvious that a global economy was the most efficient kind, and the more global the economy, the more efficient it would be.

As it turns out, none of these assumptions were correct.

Not long after I began seeking answers to these kinds of questions, I found a pamphlet lying on a campus stairway that had apparently been left by a vegetarian activist. Splashed across every page were images of hogs and chickens suffering broken bones and snipped-off beaks in filthy, cramped conditions on their way to slaughter. The headline read, "Even if you love meat, you can stop this cruelty." The text urged me to stop eating animals, or at least to cut back, to save a few of these creatures from brutality. I'd just had my first exposure to CAFOs: concentrated animal feeding operations. Until I picked up this pamphlet, I'd had no idea that my family's meat was produced this way.

Perhaps like most people, though, after this first encounter, I backed away from the cognitive dissonance these images created in my brain, unconsciously denounced the writers of the pamphlet as extremist wackos, and went home to my usual lunch of chicken tenders. But the images in the pamphlet never left me.

I began to read more about the economics of food production. I read a CNN.com article by reporter Tracie McMillan that claimed American farmers make about sixteen cents of every dollar we spend on food, which led me to the inevitable next question: who makes the other eighty-four cents? I discovered a report from the Physicians Committee for Responsible Medicine claiming that 63 percent of government farm subsidies went to the meat and dairy industries, 20 percent to grain production, and *less than 1 percent* to fruits and vegetables. No wonder a cheeseburger costs less than a salad.

To bring these ideas across with examples from the real world, I introduced my college students to an exercise called The Real Cost of Industrial Food: I brought in an assortment of processed foods from the grocery store, arranged my students in groups of four, and asked them to analyze the items for their hidden costs. They had to count the miles all the ingredients had traveled, add in the infrastructure costs of each manufacturing process, and tally the government subsidies for each item that used taxpayer dollars to reduce the item's retail price.

I had encouraged the students to get on the phone with the manufacturers of these foods and ask questions: "Good morning, I have a can of your clam chowder here. Could you tell me where your clams come from?" To put it mildly, they didn't get the reception from these companies that I'd expected. One student called to ask a soup company about their chicken, and they hung up on her. When asked where and how their hogs were raised, a canned ham company insisted on taking the student's name, address, and phone number, before responding curtly, "We obtain our hams from … *various reliable sources.*"

Why all the secrecy? After all, these manufacturers had placed their 800 numbers on their labels. Didn't they *want* to talk to people about their products?

The High Cost of Cheap Beef

We Americans love our beef. It's synonymous with manliness, wholesomeness, and prosperous middle-class eating. But since the post-World War II economic boom, our relationship to this all-American food has changed. We've come to expect our beef to be inexpensive and plentiful. Yet most of us are unaware of the hidden costs of our "cheap beef" addiction.

Because people usually buy what's cheapest, businesses must be on the lookout for ways to reduce production costs. One way to keep profits up is to drive wages down. Many meat processors employ unskilled immigrants with few other options. Working conditions are so dangerous in many meat-packing facilities that the international advocacy group Human Rights Watch has declared that the industry itself is in violation of basic human rights.

Most of us aren't aware of the social problems created by cheap beef because they seldom occur in our own communities where we can see them. A social problem that remains abstract is one we don't have to do anything about. For the near future at least, as long as we can still gnaw on a stick of jerky for less than a buck, we'll likely dismiss the plight of the beef industry worker as somebody else's problem.

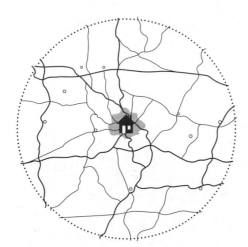

How Local Is Local?

For the purposes of this book, we'll refer to local food as any food grown within a hundred miles of your home.

Food became the common thread in the fabric of my inquiry into the future. As I ventured deeper into the issue of the American food supply and the problems that plague it, I began to understand that the main obstacle to solving the problems is that we keep trying to treat a complex issue as though it's a simple one. The decision about what to eat isn't a question of nutrition, flavor, cost, health, safety, environmental impact, or social advocacy. It's all of these at once—and more. Many voices are joining the discussion about food, but very few are speaking of it in the full knowledge that all of these issues are intertwined.

I had been marinated in food ads for so long that their effect on me had gone unnoticed. I heard so many conflicting stories on the news about diet research and health fads. The more I examined what I was hearing, the more I began to question it. Are convenience foods really more convenient? Is that artificial fruit drink with added vitamin C really as good for me as a real fruit juice? Is organic really healthier? Is nonorganic really cheaper? Will my kids rebel if I start feeding them produce instead of microwave pizza?

I decided that if I really wanted to find the answers to these questions, I'd have to use myself as a guinea pig. My husband, Al, joined in, and then my two teenage sons, Ben and Phillip, agreed to be part of the experiment, though not without a few caveats. In all the chapters that follow, I'll share the results of our experiments with fruits, vegetables, meats, dairy, baked goods, and a host of other edibles that never saw the inside of a grocery store.

In his book *The Omnivore's Dilemma*, Michael Pollan interviewed Virginia grass farmer Joel Salatin, who told him that the way he produces a chicken "is an extension of my worldview." In anthropology, a worldview is a set of assumptions about the way the world works, or should work. My reading of this was that, in harnessing his work to his worldview, Mr. Salatin had transformed his daily occupation into a statement about his place in the universe.

I loved that idea. I loved it so much I started trying to see whether it applied to any parts of my own life.

"The way I teach a class is an extension of my worldview." Yes, that's true! My work life is in sync with my picture of reality.

"The way I raise my kids is an extension of my worldview." Yes, that one works, too! The way I talk to my sons, the quantity and quality of time I spend with them, the activities we do, the expectations I have of them, the values I promote—they're all on track with my beliefs. I made a decision before they were born to stay at home with them. I worked from my home office as an editor and writer-for-hire in order to make this happen. In the grand battle between at-home moms and working moms, I was an equal opportunity offender. But I succeeded in giving my kids the kind of start I wanted for them.

"The kind of partner I am to my husband is an extension of my worldview." Yes again, although I have to give credit where it's due. Almost everything I know about being a good mate I learned from him.

"The way I drive a car is an extension of my worldview." No, that one doesn't work. I'm still driving a gas-guzzling minivan, and until the kitchen renovation is paid for and karate lessons are done, that probably won't change. The most I can do for now is to lay the groundwork for the changes I can make in the future: buy a hybrid car, teach online, maybe open a business someplace I can walk to. I'm working on it.

"The way I eat is an extension of my worldview." Well, it is *now*. Only a few years ago, it most certainly wasn't. This is where the idea for this book was born, from the journey I undertook to bring what was on my plate in line with what was in my heart.

How did I begin to break a lifelong obsession with potato chips, cookies, chicken wings, and candy bars? By knowing that I already have something in my fridge at home that's better than any of these. After forty-eight years of overeating, this is the only thing that has ever worked for me.

'll give you an example of the way this affects me on a daily basis. Today, as I left class, the thought occurred to me: It's payday. I could get some french fries. All my life, a thought like that would have been followed by an insatiable craving that built like a tidal wave until I could have chewed my way through the plate glass of the storefront to get at those greasy, golden, salt-bejeweled nuggets of pleasure.

But now, I think of the glass bottles of milk from grass-fed cows, the biscuits I'm going to bake from lovingly chosen farmers' market ingredients, the zucchini I'll sauté in garlic, and the fresh cilantro I could pick from my own garden to garnish them. Then I go home and eat the healthy, whole foods waiting for me there because I know there's nothing in any fast food restaurant in my city that's half as good as what's in my own home.

Now and again I still do get a craving for fried, salty, crunchy stuff, though not as often as I used to. But, with my new thinking, if it absolutely has to be crisp, golden, drenched in grease, and encrusted with salt, I don't

Worldview

A set of assumptions held by an individual or group about the way things are.

Five Things I Bet You Didn't Know You Could Make at Home

Breakfast cereal
Pasta
Potato chips
Sushi
Tempura

automatically think that it's something I have to purchase from a fast food joint.

When the craving shot through me today, I thought, what is it I *really* want? Some kind of potato-type thing fried to a crisp in boiling oil and bristling with salt. Then I realized, I have potatoes at home. I have oil. I have salt. I have a pot and a stove. What if I *made* french fries? *Can* I make french fries? I decided to find out.

It turns out, I could. They were salty, hot, dripping in oil—everything I needed them to be.

The difference between this homemade snack and the one I could have bought from a fast food restaurant is that this one took time and effort. When you cook most of your own food, you have to be pretty serious about wanting it. It puts an end to eating on a whim.

Producing the meal yourself shifts some of the emphasis from the eating to the cooking. Enjoying a meal doesn't have to begin and end with the time it spends in your mouth. It can begin with the planning, segue to the prepping, then cooking, plating, and on through the savoring, straight through to the *ahhhhhh* uttered over the post-meal cup of coffee. The only time during a meal like that in which calories are involved is the part in the middle when you're eating!

The rapture that real food brings is a different kind of joy. It's the jubilation of colors and textures, and the vibrancy of growing things. I pick up a bundle of massive Swiss chard leaves, the ruby veins running everywhere like rivulets of wine, and I feel the power of the earth and the potency of green and growing things, the energy of the sun, and the greatness of the cosmos.

The long, drawn-out love affair of the heart, soul, and senses you can have with a home-cooked feast is very different from the casual experience of a peel-the-lid, nuke-and-eat meal. It is far longer, far deeper. There's not only the intense blush of first discovery when you spy those voluptuous leaves in the produce case and first hold them in your hands. There's the rush of acquisition, the bringing them home, the finding a place for them in the kitchen.

I'm in love with dark leafy greens: the crinkled kale, the leathery elephant-ears of collards, and the chard with its veins in a carnival of colors. The leaves I buy in a given week fill an entire refrigerator shelf by themselves. The midsection of our fridge looks like darkest Africa.

Then comes the cooking: the careful washing, trimming, and placing in boiling water; the choosing of other ingredients, herbs, and sauces to

Refrigerator Feng Shui: Arranging Your Fridge to Accommodate Fresh Local Food

Your fresh leafy greens will be the first to wither, so keep them in a crisper or lidded container, but make sure they stay where you can see them so you remember to cook them.

Set aside a large bowl or bin for hard fruits and vegetables: apples, pears, peppers, zucchinis, cucumbers, and the like. They can cohabitate without bruising one another.

Prepare a similar bowl or bin for softies such as eggplants and oranges. Don't put tomatoes or avocados in the fridge.

Fresh herbs, asparagus, and celery keep longest if you cut off their bottoms and place them upright in a jar of cold water. Change the water every few days.

Keep cheeses as airtight as you can. Freeze any meats you won't use within three days.

Some vegetables are hardy enough to sit in a decorative bowl or basket on your counter: onions and winter squashes can pretty up your kitchen while they wait to be devoured. Potatoes will store a while, but keep them in a cool dark place so they don't turn green and poisonous.

---

complement. Unusable leaf tips or stems seem too precious to throw away. They go out to the compost pile so that their fertility enriches next year's garden.

As the food cooks, there's the anticipation, the apprehension. I want it to turn out right. It's all drama and suspense. When I'm cooking, time stops. I'm pure concentration, checking, tasting, adding, twiddling knobs, muttering. I'm fully in the now. I've caught my husband watching me do this, an amused smile on his face. Few other parts of my life allow the pure focus I find in the kitchen.

When I put effort into a meal, I make sure everyone sits down at the table together to eat. I want to watch their faces as they taste it. I wait for that flush of pride when they go back for seconds and thirds. It's satisfying in a way few other things in life are: knowing I fed my family well, knowing they loved the food I made for them.

There's simply far more joy to be had, eating this way. It's not a Hoover-it-down way to get full fast, but a sensual, communal, and spiritual act of love. It's less like a mechanical act and more like a romance.

Next comes joy on a different level. To eat the gifts of Earth, in almost exactly the form Earth delivered them, gives me a feeling of deep connection to nature. It makes me feel like I'm part of it all: the energy streaming from

Five Things to Tell Your Kids Before You Turn Them Loose in the Kitchen

1. Wash the potatoes.
2. Yes, you really do have to take the time to cut off the inedible parts.
3. Don't put salad in the freezer.
4. Yes, it is possible for food to be both raw *and* burnt at the same time.
5. Cooking dinner is not compatible with watching *Star Trek* reruns. If in doubt about this point, see number 4.

Top Ten Reasons to Buy Local Food

1. Buying locally gives you the opportunity to involve yourself directly with the source of your food.
2. Local farmers are more transparent about their food production methods.
3. Local farmers are part of your community. They have more reason to be accountable to you.
4. Local farms are likely to be diversified, so they make less of an impact on their environment.
5. Local farms are more likely to use environmentally friendly techniques.
6. Local food hasn't traveled hundreds or thousands of miles. By eating it, you're conserving fossil fuels.
7. Local food is usually grown from varieties suited to your climate, so they make more efficient use of resources.
8. Local food is likely to be less processed—better for your health and that of the planet.
9. Fresh food retains more of its nutrients.
10. Fresh food tastes better, and local food is the freshest.

the sun, the minerals enriching the earth, the rainfall, the burrowing roots sucking it all up, all that goodness coursing into the leaves, then through our bodies.

Even that's not where the pleasure ends. There's also joy that comes from knowing that my actions are in harmony with my values. By choosing one food system over another, I'm not exploiting underpaid workers, adding toxic waste to waterways, or strip-mining the future. By careful, conscious eating, I'm helping to maintain life cycles and soils, supporting farmers who caretake the land.

Oh yes, there's one more pleasure, one that I'm still in the midst of discovering: the joy of taking care of *myself*. When I eat like this, I eat not just to fulfill a need in the moment, but to hedge my bets for a longer, happier future. After switching from processed artificial food to the real thing, my thoughts are coming to me clearer and cleaner. My energy level has stopped taking its usual roller-coaster ride. Instead, I now enjoy a smooth, cool burn that propels me through the entire day.

Now that I'm healthier, I can look forward to a future that's more fulfilling than my past, one in which I can quit taking blood pressure medicines, dance the evening away with my sexy husband, and sleep soundly through the night. When I take care of myself this well, I begin to believe that I'm worth taking care of. It's nicer to go through my days that way than it is to eat like I'm not worth the effort. And I can make that empowering choice three times a day!

What began with visits to local farms and a few cautious kitchen experiments grew into a full-on passion for alternatives to industrial food. I want to share this journey with you, as intimately as I can. This journey has been a source of intense pleasure and deep satisfaction. Nothing sold at the mall, broadcast on cable TV, or downloaded from the Internet could ever possibly compare to the soul-saturating *rapture* of eating a tomato that tastes like it came from my granddaddy's backyard, or baking my first batch of homemade biscuits and watching my family wolf them down.

You may decide to opt into local food for the health benefits, the economic fair play, or the good of the environment. But first and foremost, do it for the bliss it will bring you!

Roasted Butternut Squash

Butternut squash is quite possibly one of the most delicious foods in the entire world, and it's at its best when served solo. It's a great way to introduce your family to the concept of eating whole, fresh veggies that have had hardly anything done to them and which, consequently, taste like what they really are:

1 large butternut squash

1/4 cup olive oil

1/4 teaspoon nutmeg

Preheat oven to 400 degrees.

Pour the olive oil into a large casserole dish so that the bottom is coated. Slice the neck of the squash into 1/2-inch medallions, then slice each medallion in half. Revel in the sensuous sunset-orange color of the vegetable. Slice the bottom part in half lengthwise and scoop out the seeds (rinse and place these on a pie plate for drying if you're a gardener), then cut into quarter-inch slices. This part of the vegetable will make little crescent moon shapes.

Rub each piece in the oil at the bottom of the casserole dish, then flip it over so that both sides are oiled. Sprinkle each piece lightly with nutmeg. Roast until tender and lightly toasted, about 10 to 15 minutes.

You can serve the slices with the skin still on. Or, after cooking, you can peel the skin away nicely with just a fork.

2

Feeding Your Worldview

How to Use This Book

Three things cannot be long hidden: the sun, the moon, and the truth. —*Buddha*

When we talk about economic systems, my anthropology students do an exercise called A Day Without. They pick one item from a list of things that they're used to taking for granted, such as gasoline, electricity, electronics, plastics, or processed food. On day one, they track their usage of that item. Then, on day two, they try to give it up, cold turkey, for twenty-four hours.

It's an eye-opener, for me and for them. One student who tried to do without plastics discovered that he couldn't use his kitchen trash can because it had a plastic bag in it. He ended up throwing his trash on the floor for the rest of the day. His mom loved me for that assignment. Another student got her whole family in on the exercise. They shut off the electricity in their house for twenty-four hours and called it a disaster-preparedness drill. They were on an electrically powered well, so they ended up having to borrow forty gallons of water from the neighbor just to flush their toilets. A student who gave up electronics went to a party that night and, while exchanging phone numbers with a girl he'd met, discovered that he couldn't use his phone to take her number. Instead, he wrote it down on a napkin. The girl thought this was so cute that she called him the next day for a date!

About half the students choose processed food for their day without, maybe because it seems easy. Those who tackle this one usually end up blowing it long before the day is over. A few can't find more than one or two nonprocessed food in their homes and go through the day noshing on nothing but carrots. In their papers, they tell me they never realized just how much they had been drawn in by the convenience, how dependent on it they had become. Nearly all of the students who survive their day-long abstinence from processed foods report that, although it wasn't easy, they did feel a lot better the next day. Quite a few of them declare that they've decided to eat like that more often!

I'm hoping that this book will bring a similar kind of *"aha"* for you. At first, it might seem as though eating locally involves giving things up, but it's really about taking new things on. In letting go of the habits that cheap and convenient foods have engendered in us, we're opening ourselves up to a world of new discoveries. You're not losing the foods you enjoy; you're gaining a new way of relating to your nourishment that will offer you whole new dimensions of pleasure, health, satisfaction, and peace.

Eating to Satisfy Your Worldview

This is definitely *not* a diet book. It's not a nutritional manual. Neither is it a cookbook, a list of rules about eating, a collection of cute gardening anecdotes, or an agricultural manifesto. I tried to create this book so that it would be multifaceted, rather than one-dimensional, because I think that's part of our problem, as a nation of eaters. We seem to be able to think in only one direction at a time. This year, we're convinced that omega-3s will be the key to saving our health. A few years ago, it was the low-carb diet, and before that, flax. In the 1980s, oat bran enjoyed a good long stint as the miracle food. We tend to treat even complex subjects like diet and nutrition as though they have singular, one-size-fits-all solutions.

The reality is that there's much more to the act of eating than the nourishment we derive from a single nutrient. In fact, there's far more to ingesting food than the simple act of nourishing ourselves. Eating is also a political act, an economic activity, a bonding ritual, a cultural statement, and an interaction with the natural world.

To illustrate this idea, let's take a mental snapshot of the act of eating. There's you, about to enjoy your first bite of that cheese tortellini you brought for lunch. Zoom in on the moment that fork touches your lips. Suppose we freeze that image, right there. Now, let's rewind.

Where was that tortellini before it came to you? Before it landed on your plate, the pasta had to be cooked by someone. Was it a loved one, who did it because feeding you lunch was an expression of their bond with you, or

Processed foods

Foods that have been significantly altered from their natural state, especially because of numerous industrial processes. Foods with a high content of artificially produced ingredients. Foods that are designed and manufactured in an industrial setting to compete with other similar products in the commercial food marketplace.

A Holistic View of Local Food Issues

Choosing to eat food from local sources is not just a matter of health or flavor, but also of safety, community and family cohesion, local and international economics, human equality, environmental conservation, and more.

was it a restaurant employee, a stranger, motivated primarily by economic gain? Where did the flour come from? How many miles has it traveled to get to you? By what means was it grown? Did it enrich or deplete its ecosystem? The cheese inside the pasta, did it come from a cow that spends her days being milked mechanically and fed an unnatural diet of corn? Or does she feed at will on grass and mosey into the barn to be milked by people who call her by name?

Okay, let's return to the present, that freeze-frame, fork-to-lips snapshot. Now we'll go forward into the future. You bite into your tortellini. You savor. You swallow. Does it satisfy? Will it give you long-lasting, clean-burning energy? Does it nourish your body, or was the sole reason for eating it the ten seconds of pleasure it created on your tongue? Along with the carbs, protein, and nutrients that you probably did want, did it add things to your body that you'd rather *not* have? If you eat mostly food like this for the next several decades of your life, what will be the cumulative effect on your health?

Now, back to that snapshot. There you are again, with the tortellini poised on the tip of your tongue. This time, let's pull back to the panoramic view around you. We see that you're enjoying your lunch in suburban, middle-class America in the early years of the twenty-first century. You're eating your second meal of three, after a good breakfast, with a full dinner to look forward to at the end of the day. You're accustomed to eating this way. You've never gone to bed at night without knowing where your food will come from tomorrow. Yet, you're fully aware that millions of people in the world aren't as fortunate as you. This fact often leaves you feeling that you want to do something to fix that situation, something real, though you're not certain what that might be.

You're also aware that there are larger issues related to food that hit closer to home than this. Let's assume for a moment that you bought that tortellini in a package at the grocery store and you cooked it yourself. In that case, Uncle Sam is picking up the tab for a large part of your meal. The U.S. government pays hefty subsidies to large industrial wheat and dairy producers, but very few to small family-operated ones. So by buying this kind of pasta, from this source, you've encouraged one kind of agricultural economy and discouraged another.

Now, let's pull the focus back even further, to the whole world. The agricultural practices that produced your lunch, and the infrastructure and energy that it took to bring it to you, had an impact on the natural systems of Earth. Was it a positive one? Or did you unwittingly add to a problem that may lead us into an ecological tailspin?

Okay, back to you and your tortellini. As you take that bite, you're aware that eating is not a singular, isolated act, but a complex behavior with larger implications. Your food choices have a history, a future, and a place in the larger world. The act of consuming food can't be divorced from health, nutrition, agriculture, economy, energy production, ecology, global social issues, environmentalism, and probably a host of other issues we haven't thought of yet. Viewed this way, that single act of eating takes on a new importance.

One of the marvelous aspects of the twenty-first century, with its global society, is that we now have a chance to see the impact of our worldviews on the big picture. More than any other time in the history of our kind, we can recognize that our actions have consequences. To live in harmony with your worldview is, in Gandhi's words, to "be the change you want to see in the world." In a small, quiet, powerful way, we can help to create the kind of society we'd like to live in by the choices that we make, even when it comes to an act as seemingly innocuous as eating.

You might have an impulse to argue with this idea. You may be thinking, "I'm only one person, out of about 317 million in the United States, seven *billion* worldwide. Against numbers like those, the impact of one person's actions is too small to measure." You might conclude from this line of thinking that it doesn't matter what you do. But you'd be mistaken. Each of us has only our own actions—no less, no more—with which to affect the world.

Besides, if you think that you're acting in a vacuum, you've missed one of the fundamental traits of humankind: our interconnectedness. People see the things you do, the choices you make. If you're flourishing, if your choices are bringing you joy, you'll attract people. They'll want to know your secret. If the reasons you give for the things you do make sense to them, you may influence their choices. Never underestimate the power of a thoughtful, loving soul living happily according to his or her worldview.

How Do You Come to Me?

I'm assuming that you've come to this book already convinced. You may have read books such as Michael Pollan's *Omnivore's Dilemma*, Eric Schlosser's *Fast Food Nation*, and John Robbins's *Food Revolution*. You may have seen movies such as *Fed Up*; *Food, Inc.*; or *Supersize Me*. You've decided

Industrial Food

Food that has been grown by industrial agriculture and processed for the commercial marketplace through a highly mechanized system of mass production designed to maximize profit by producing large quantities of uniform products at as low a cost as possible.

Is All Industrial Food Bad? Is All Local Food Good?

To say that the industrial food system is "broken" is not to suggest that the whole thing must be scrapped. Industrial agriculture has contributed to the availability and security of food worldwide. What is "broken" is the link between producer and consumer that would allow for informed choices. Eating locally is a way to begin examining America's food production systems, because this is the food whose provenance we can readily access.

you want to eat differently, and what you need now is some practical information about how to act on that decision. You've got the *why*. Now you're seeking the *what, where, how,* and *what to expect*.

I'm also thinking that you're starting this journey from deep within the industrial food system, just as I did. You're accustomed to eating at fast food restaurants and buying your groceries from large supermarkets. You're not, at the moment, in the habit of cooking a lot of meals at home. In fact, you might even be convinced that you *can't* cook, or that putting home-cooked dinners on your family's table every night will mean a lot of unpleasant drudgery. You might even be so new to the idea of buying whole, fresh, locally grown foods that you're not sure what you would do with an entire butternut squash or a whole chicken. You've probably heard that this kind of food is so expensive that a shift to buying local food is impractical. You're apprehensive, in half a dozen ways, about making changes to something as fundamental as your eating habits.

That's okay. You're not alone. My family and I worked our way through these issues. Throughout the book, I'll share our experiences, and perhaps I can help you take a shortcut past some of our screwups and profit from our mistakes.

How Do I Come to You?

I come to you first as a fellow eater, suburbanite, and mom, trying to make the best choices that I can for myself and my family, and trying to live what I believe. Most of what I have to share with you, I'll frame from this perspective.

In this book, I'm not coming to you as a professional, but as a friend and neighbor, sharing an experience and hoping you'll find it useful. Now and again I'll tap into my background in sociocultural anthropology, because it really does have a lot to say on the subject of food.

There are surely plenty of people with more experience in the local food movement than I have. I can't claim to be an expert on it. What I have to offer you are my experiences as a local eater, in the hope that, if you're on a similar path, some of what I've been through may be helpful.

What to Expect When You Switch to Local Food

If you're serious about changing from an all-industrial diet to a lifestyle of mostly local whole foods, you're in for a bigger change than you realize.

We're not just talking about eating the same stuff as before, but from local sources. In many cases, you'll be eating totally different foods. Making this switch will affect other aspects of your life.

For instance, cooking and eating will probably become a more central part of your daily routine, will occupy more of your time, and will become a deeply social activity. Your hobbies will change. Cooking will probably become one of them, and maybe gardening, too. You'll spend more time pulling out weeds and less time pulling out your wallet. You'll take the kids to visit local farms instead of theme parks. You'll spend more of your time under green canopies and less under golden arches.

You may find that your energy level increases, so you may become more active. You may start placing a higher value on nature. You'll get excited over things that other people just don't find as stimulating: dirt, worms, kitchen scraps, and animal excrement. If you're like me, you'll start talking back to your television, telling those industrial food advertisers just what you think of their products.

Here's one change you might not be expecting: your taste for foods may evolve quite a lot, and much faster than you'd think. In the years that I've been eating local food, I've been amazed at how my tastes have changed. I've broken lifelong addictions without even trying. If you told me three years ago that I would lose my craving for diet soda, I'd have said you were out of your mind. But as I got used to the vibrant taste of real food, I became sensitive to the flavor of chemicals in the processed kind. Similarly, I used to call myself a protein junkie. For me, it wasn't a proper meal without a slab of meat at its center. But I discovered that fresh vegetables, well prepared, not only taste as savory as any meat, but also give me cleaner energy and a clearer mind, not to mention a happier doctor when I go in for my blood pressure checks.

My family and I still have a weakness for processed crunchies—potato chips, crackers, sweetened cereal—but it's not as bad as it was before. One Saturday morning, my husband gave in to a moment of temporary insanity and brought home not one but *two* boxes of a popular brand of sugar-laden, highly processed breakfast cereal we both had known and loved from childhood. He and my sons devoured the first box in the time it took me to drive

A Note About the Recipes

At the end of each chapter, you'll find a simple recipe that can be made with mostly local, whole foods. These are dishes that my husband, sons, and I have cooked since our experiment with local food began, definitely *not* high cuisine. They're either our own creations, simplified versions of other recipes, or in a few cases, attempts to recreate childhood favorites from memory. They're not meant to be fancy or professional; rather, the opposite. They're simple, easy, and hopefully a fun way to ease into a new style of eating.

home from my morning class. But the *second* box, miraculously, remained untouched for nearly a week.

That the second box sat unravaged for so long shows just how far we've come. A year ago, the second box would have met the same fate as the first, and I would have been one of the main causes. This time, I wasn't even tempted.

But if I *had* given in to temptation, how bad would it have been, really? I've decided to forgive myself for slip-ups. It doesn't help to beat myself up. So if a little crunchy decadence brings you joy, and your worldview is happy with most of the other choices you've made, can you give yourself a break now and again?

House Rules

Most of the local food producers I've met practice transparency of method, so I'd like to do the same. I want take a moment to lay out a few of the operating rules for this book.

First, I'm deliberately putting this subject on a positive footing. I'm not anti-anything, but I'm pro quite a bit. I'm not anti-industrial foods; I'm pro local-sustainable foods. I'm not anti-fast food; I'm pro home-cooked food. I'm not anti-supermarkets; I'm pro a wide variety of food sources. I'm not anti-meat; I'm pro people having the right information to make choices that affect their health. I'm not even anti-GMOs (genetically modified organisms), but I'm pro labeling them as such. I'm not seeking to run anyone out of business or cause anyone harm. I don't have an ax to grind or a score to settle. I just want to see everyone well fed and living within our planet's carrying capacity. If we can just do that, there isn't a single other problem of human existence that we can't solve.

Second, I don't want to wear a label, and I don't want you to, either. So let's make an agreement: no name-calling. My colleague Arlene, a college instructor who is passionate about making sure everyone on the planet has access to clean water, once told me that her in-laws have labeled her a hippie peacenik. Why the name-calling? That old "sticks and stones" song from childhood is wrong. Names do hurt. You don't call someone a peacenik to show her respect. But really, what's wrong with advocating for peace? Who could possibly object to that?

Like Arlene, I don't want to be pigeonholed or labeled. Like any other human being, I'm a bit too complex to be well represented by a label. I don't want to be called a busybody, foodie, greenie, hippie, bleeding-heart liberal, Luddite, or anything else. I don't want to be called anti-God, anti-America, or anti-capitalist, especially because, in truth, I'm none of these things; rather the opposite, in fact. I love my country, I admire people of sincere faith, and I appreciate the freedom I have to make a living, support my family, and live as I choose. I'm here to learn, and I'm freely admitting my ignorance. I'll ask you to respect me and all others who are trying to make the best we can out of what comes to us.

Even if you read what's here and decide *not* to make any changes to your food life, that's okay too. It doesn't mean you're my enemy, or that I'm yours. After more than a few decades of living, I've come to understand that if someone makes a different choice than I do, that doesn't have to threaten me or make me feel as though I need to win that individual over. I can respect someone who makes a different choice.

I don't want to start an argument or make anyone angry. Food is a touchy subject, although I'm not entirely sure why. I understand that people feel very strongly about environmentalism. Others feel very protective about their food traditions and what they view as the American way of life. Many people view a critical examination of something they hold dear as a threat, or they feel that to find fault with any of it is to condemn all of it. This is not my intent.

We're not going to do black-and-white, either/or, good-or-bad thinking here. We're just looking to make small improvements where we can. If someone makes a slight change for the better, it doesn't help to condemn him for not making a total change for the best.

I've already had a certain amount of hatred thrown my way, just by teaching a subject that puts all humankind on an equal footing and positions us solidly as part of the natural world. Once, a student directly threatened me with violence. The college politely removed him from my classroom. Another student wrote on his evaluation, "May God have mercy on your soul." None of this has stopped me.

Will you see hypocrisy in some of what I say and do? If you want to see it, you will, but I hope you won't be trying to. The potential to appear hypocritical is present in all of us because we're complicated and imperfect, and any aspect of our behavior could be interpreted in all kinds of ways.

How This Book is Organized

I've arranged this book to be as user-friendly as possible. You can start here and read straight to the end of the book, or you can home in on the specific chapters and sections you need at a given time.

The book has four parts. Part I gives you the basics and frames the issue. You've probably already read Chapter 1, the story of how we fell in love with local food. You're just now finishing Chapter 2, which shows you what to expect from the book. Chapter 3 provides you with a solid overview of local food: what it is, who grows it, and what it is that makes it so special. Chapter 4 puts the current state of our industrial food system into a historical context.

Part II is filled with practical information, news you can use. Chapter 5 introduces you to some terms you've probably heard that may have boggled you, such as "organic," "free range," and "all natural." It will help you sort the good stuff from the bad. Chapter 6 gives you a side-by-side comparison of local foods next to their industrial counterparts. Chapter 7 shows you where to go to find great local food, from food co-ops to consumer supported agriculture (CSAs) and more. Chapter 8 will let you in on a few secrets that could have you eating some of the best food in the world and actually paying less for it than you used to at the supermarket.

Part III focuses on the changes in your lifestyle that are likely to occur as a result of your shift to a new way of eating. Chapter 9 helps you figure out what to do with this glorious stuff when you get it home. If you're staring down your first whole chicken or mound of Swiss chard, this chapter will give you a heads-up about cooking with the real thing. Chapter 10 explains why eating locally means eating seasonally. It explains why local eaters don't dine on peaches in February, and why seasonal eating actually provides more pleasure than devouring anything you want whenever you want it. Chapter 11 will introduce you to the ultimate in local food, the kind that comes from your own backyard. If you're considering growing some of your own, you'll find some tips on getting started. Chapter 12 helps you troubleshoot your new lifestyle: how to find time to snap green beans, whether eating locally means an end to dining out, and if you can expect the local food diet to show up on your favorite daytime talk show as the newest weight loss miracle.

Part IV of the book addresses the bigger picture: the impact you will be making on your world by adopting this new way of eating. Chapter 13 details the reasons why this way of eating strengthens the bonds between families

Locavore

A person who obtains most of her food from sources within a hundred-mile radius of her home.

and communities. Chapter 14 explains local food from an ecological point of view, how this kind of eating puts you in sync with the way that nature tends to do things. If you've ever wondered at the phrase, "nature doesn't make trash," this chapter will explain that the natural world operates in mutually reinforcing, holistic systems. Chapter 15 places the issue of local food in a global perspective and explains how supporting locally owned production worldwide can help us move smoothly through the next few decades of socioeconomic transition. Finally, Chapter 16 offers support for responding to the people who will want to call you colorful names and throw negativity your way simply because of the food choices you've made. Don't think they won't.

You Make the Change, I'll Support You

If "how do I feed my worldview?" is the central question of this book, variety is the central answer. Instead of assuming there's a single way to accomplish this, let's look for as many variations on the theme as we can.

You know your own life best. You're better qualified than I am to decide which of these alternatives work for you and your family. Throughout this book, I'll give you as many options and perspectives as I can, and you can choose the ones that make the most sense for your unique circumstances.

Sound like a plan?

Southwestern Twice-Baked Potatoes

8 medium potatoes

1 pound ground turkey or beef (optional)

1 cup black beans

1/2 cup corn

1 large onion, diced

1 large pepper, diced

1 teaspoon chili powder

1/2 teaspoon powdered chipotle pepper

4 ounces cheddar cheese

Bake potatoes at 400 degrees until soft. Slice in half and scoop out an indentation in each half. Sauté onion, corn, and pepper. Add beans, meat, and powders. Sauté until meat is cooked. Mound sautéed mix into each potato half. Bake ten minutes. Top with cheddar cheese and bake five more minutes. Serves four.

3

What Is Local Food?

And What Is So Darn Great About It?

Before eating, always take time to thank the food. —*Arapaho proverb*

For Thanksgiving dinner, we roasted a dinosaur.

That's how it seemed at the time. Weighing in at twenty-four pounds, he was the biggest turkey I'd ever seen.

Our enormous Mister Tom was a Bourbon Red, a once-common historic breed that only a handful of farmers raise today. He came from Nick's Organic Farm in Adamstown, Md., twenty minutes from our house. Nick Maravell's farm raises Angus cattle and organic grains along with chickens, turkeys, and eggs. We had visited the farm during an open house in October and had seen our bird while he was still alive, although we didn't know at the time which one he was.

He and his companions sported cherry-red wattles dangling below their slate-blue bald pates and rows of copper-and-cream feathers. They gobbled in rhythm. A few seconds of silence would pass with nothing but the synchronized bobbing of blue heads, and then, simultaneously, they'd take up a melodious, liquid warbling before quieting down again. I couldn't tell who started it, or why. But they seemed to be doing it *happily*.

These birds had a good life, that much was clear. Owner Nick Maravell told our visiting group that the turkeys were moved to a fresh patch of pasture about once a week. They ate organic feed grown on site, along with, Nick explained, an occasional swig of milk from the farm's two Guernsey cows. No antibiotics, no hormones. They lived days of breezy sunshine and tall grass, securely netted off from predators, with plenty of room to move about and exude their regal turkeyness.

When Mister Tom's number was up, he ended his days in the same place he began them, possibly without having the slightest inkling that he had died. I didn't watch them do it, but I saw the equipment and read about the process by which it was done.

When we picked him up the day before Thanksgiving, he still looked like a bird, minus the head, feet, and feathers. My husband, Al, drove to four different stores to find a pan big enough to roast him. We brined our bird with kosher salt and vegetable stock overnight, then, Thanksgiving morning, slathered him in olive oil and sage and shoehorned him into the oven. The creature took more than nine hours to cook. When he was done, we served him to our family, who showered us with compliments and happily took home tubs of leftovers. Weeks later, they were still texting us, wanting to know what we had done to make our turkey taste so good.

We hadn't done anything out of the ordinary, except to purchase him locally.

Before we get much further into this discussion about local food, we'd better define our terms. Our national craving for sustenance that doesn't reek heavily of a corporation is known by many names, but it's most often called the local food movement. There's a lot more to local food, of course, than simply the fact that it was grown someplace near the person who eats it, but the word "local" is a shorthand way to describe it.

The people who adopt this way of eating are seeking food that was grown close enough to where they live that it hasn't burned buckets of fossil fuel to get to them. They want to know that it was produced in a way that doesn't deplete resources or damage its ecosystem. They care about the well-being of animals raised for human consumption and want to be assured that these creatures live cruelty-free lives. They would like to feel confident that what they consume isn't laden with suspicious chemicals and isn't likely to make them sick. They want food that isn't processed beyond all recognition. These are the overt reasons people usually offer as their explanation for making this change in their food-buying habits.

But there are other, somewhat intangible reasons for this shift, and these too need to be added to the mix in order to get a full picture of what local food is really about. It's also about food that is honestly priced, and that at the same time earns an abundant living for the people who produce it. It's about food that is equally available to all, helping to move us toward a world

What Brings You to Local Food?

WHAT ARE YOUR CONCERNS?		HOW IS LOCAL FOOD A FACTOR?
Health	Obesity, diseases of affluence, asthma, diabetes	Local whole foods are less processed, fresher.
Safety	Food-borne illnesses, genetically modified organisms (GMOs), chemicals	Local foods have shorter distribution chains. Some small local producers avoid GMOs. Some use no artificial inputs.
Nutrition	Fat, cholesterol, empty calories	Some small-scale production methods result in lower fat and cholesterol, more nutritional density.
Flavor	Taste, texture, freshness	Fresh foods grown in healthy soil taste best. Heirloom varieties are bred for flavor.
Animals	Cruelty, suppression of natural behaviors	Many small producers allow you to visit and see for yourself how the animals are treated.
Environment	Global warming, pollution, degradation, depletion	Some small-scale production methods focus on ecosystem health. Eating local involves less shipping and thus a smaller carbon footprint.
Family	Meals on the go, little time to spend together	Eating local encourages family meals, cooking skills, agrarian knowledge, work ethic, and social skills.
Community	Would like to know my neighbors	Interact with neighbors in community gardens, food banks. Buy from someone you know.
Local	Family businesses losing out to corporations	Local food keeps dollars in the community.
National	Social stratification, food deserts, corporate welfare	Farmers and small-scale food businesses retain more of each food dollar. Eating local reduces dependence on corporations.
Global	Poverty, exploitation, people forced off their lands	Local food supports community self-sufficiency, reduces global corporate exploitation.

in which no one goes hungry. It's also about food that enhances connections to nature, community, family, and friends.

The common thread that unites all these motives is *awareness*. Today, many people are discovering that they haven't got a clue where their nourishment comes from, and that, in the absence of their involvement with their food's origins, much of the stuff they consume has been produced in a way that doesn't sing a harmonious tune with their conscience, their health, or their worldview. In each of these issues is the idea that *people have the right to know certain things about their food*.

To fully define what we mean by local food, let's take a look at each of these factors.

Food That Was Grown Close By

Today, more of us are realizing that we can't continue to burn as much fossil fuel as we want. We understand that excessive burning of oil and gas damages our planet's atmosphere and raises global temperatures. The consequence of this awareness is that we're looking around for ways to satisfy our wants and needs with things that are produced closer to home.

Locally produced goods don't travel as far to get to us as industrial products do, so buying them saves fuel. They're a better fit with our ecological sensibilities. Plus, whenever we buy locally, we're doing our part to support a supplier within our community, who will, we hope, be there for us in case the shipped items become astronomically expensive or are no longer available. They're one more hedge against an unknown future.

The bottom line is that, when we purchase an item, we're beginning to pay a lot more attention to the number of miles it has traveled. We're coming to realize that much of our food has logged some serious mileage to get to the store where we buy it.

Where does it come from? Much of our produce was born and raised in California. It may have traveled up to three thousand miles to reach those of us on the East Coast. Of course, not all California produce comes from massive industrial monoculture. Even if you live in California, you can choose small-scale farms rather than large ones.

We also import a great deal of our winter produce from foreign countries. Because we've grown used to having asparagus in December and grapes in February, a good bit of the fresh food we consume must come from the southern hemisphere, where the seasons are the reverse of ours. Our imported produce may have come from as far away as Argentina (it's 5,604 miles from Buenos Aires to Chicago—a city roughly in the center of the U.S.), Chile (5,320 miles from Santiago to Chicago), or New Zealand (8,203 miles from Auckland to Chicago).

Much of our beef, pork, and poultry also hails from the Midwest but, according to *Food Safety News*, several billion pounds a year are imported from Canada, Mexico, Australia, New Zealand, and Central and South American countries such as Nicaragua, Brazil, and Uruguay. A good bit of this imported beef is from cows raised on pasture that was formerly rain forest.

Most of the corn and soy that feeds our meat animals, as well as those grains that go into our breads, cereals, and processed foods, were grown in the Midwest. Nearly every U.S. state has land capable of growing cereal grains, and most states do produce some grain, but we have concentrated the growing of these grains in one area of the nation, where they are grown all by themselves ("monocultured") on a massive scale and shipped elsewhere for processing before the food products come to us. The processed foods may have made three or four journeys already before they make their way to the grocery store shelf where we find them.

The fact that our food is so remarkably well traveled is a relatively new phenomenon. Two hundred years ago, most people ate local food out of sheer necessity, because it was impossible to ship perishable items over long distances. Imported foods were for the wealthiest people, who enjoyed them as luxuries. With the advent of railroads, jets, and refrigerated containers, shipped food went from novelty to staple, and finally, to a taken-for-granted way of life.

Until recently, few people were aware that their food had traveled hundreds and thousands of miles to get to them. Even if someone mentioned that fact to them, they'd be unlikely to recognize why it was a problem.

Many futurists speculate that this nonchalance about the fuel we consume will continue until the day gas becomes too expensive to burn for anything other than necessities. Then all of us will join the local food movement, whether we want to or not.

Once a person makes the decision to start eating locally, their next question is usually, *how close is local?* How close by must food be grown in order to count? The quick and easy answer is, the closer the better (see Chapter 11, which is all about growing food in your own backyard). Closest is best not only because of the fuel saved but because the freshest produce is also most

Can Locavorism Alone Feed the Entire World?

With a global population of 7 billion and counting, not likely. A global food system provides many benefits, including a wide variety of foods and the assurance that food is available in the face of regional crises such as a droughts. Locavorism is evidence that, in any complex society, there's room for more than one system, that all systems benefit from a little variety and competition, and that consumers have a right to information and choice.

Has Your Chicken Been to China?

In September 2013, the USDA approved four Chinese poultry processing plants to ship chicken to the United States. Apparently, the chickens they'll be shipping to us are our own. That's right, we'll be shipping U.S.-raised chickens to China for processing, then they'll ship the processed meat back to us for sale here at home. Although China is a magnificent country in many respects, it doesn't have the greatest reputation for food safety.

If you want to avoid eating chicken that's traveled further abroad than you have, you might run into some difficulty, because the USDA currently doesn't require point-of-origin labeling on poultry. If you buy your chicken from a supermarket or restaurant, you have no way of knowing where it comes from. But one way you can be certain where your bird has been is to buy it from a local farmer who raised the animal himself.

nutritious and best tasting. If you don't believe me, all you have to do is try biting into a cucumber minutes after pulling it off the vine.

For a simple rule of thumb, though, food is considered local if it was grown within a hundred-mile radius of your home. It comes from the same region in which you live. It didn't need a refrigerated tractor-trailer, or a passport, to get to you.

Closer in is even better. If you get most of your sustenance from small farmers who live within a fifteen-minute drive from your home, the money you pay them is more likely to be rolled back into your community, and everybody wins.

But what if you live deep within a highly populated area and the closest thing to a farm within fifteen minutes of your house is the idyllic silo and sunny rows of wheat pictured on the cereal boxes at your grocery store? In that case, you may find that your local farmers will come to you. According to *USA Today*, in 2012, the number of U.S. Department of Agriculture-registered farmers' markets in the United States reached 7,864. Chances are good there's one near you. If you're not certain where or when your nearest farmers' market can be found, check out the section on them in Chapter 7.

How strict will you be with yourself? How locally do you have to eat to feel at peace with your conscience? That's up to you, but I believe we can allow ourselves a few little imported luxuries without wrecking the planet or exploiting anyone. If we do nothing more than concentrate on habitually eating what *can* be grown locally, we are making an important shift. If we imported only those things that can't be produced efficiently in our region, especially if we weren't in a hurry to get them and didn't mind paying what they really cost, we would be well on our way to creating a different kind of food economy.

It's mostly the I-have-to-have-it-NOW mind-set, which has become part of our culture and results in millions of gallons of fuel spent to rush imported food to us by jet. With forethought, we could buy four months' worth of olive oil, coffee, and chocolate at one time and wait for the next batch to arrive on a slow boat.

Food That Doesn't Damage or Deplete Its Environment

One of the great things about eating local food is that, on a sunny Saturday afternoon, you can literally go to the place where it's produced and see for yourself how it's grown. You can "shake the hand that feeds you," as journalist Michael Pollan puts it in his book *In Defense of Food: An Eater's Manifesto*. You have an opportunity to meet the people who produce what you eat and ask them questions. By doing this, you can collect firsthand evidence that your sustenance is grown in an environmentally sound way.

One of the really lovely things you'll discover about visiting local farms that open their doors to the public is that these farmers *want* to meet you. They like it when customers take the time to visit them and cultivate a relationship. Most of the small producers I've met are passionate about sustainable farming and love when people take an interest. They tend to place a high value on transparency: making their methods visible to the consumer. The farmers I've met are down-to-earth people who love what they do. You'll like them.

You'll also like the way they grow your food. Many small-scale producers are organic, or nearly organic. Many avoid using chemical pesticides, herbicides, and fertilizers. They shun genetically modified produce and prefer to grow heirloom varieties of fruits and vegetables, the time-tested ones ideally suited to a region and bred for their flavor. Most small-scale farmers don't routinely shoot up perfectly healthy chickens, pigs, and cattle with antibiotics because they believe animals raised well in stress-free conditions are naturally disease resistant.

The food these small producers grow takes far less of a toll on its environment, and not just because it's grown with fewer chemical inputs. Small herds and flocks leave a lighter footprint on the land than massive ones. Plus, the methods many small producers use consist of mutually enhancing systems that actually leave the land healthier than it would be in the absence of such farms. Many small-scale livestock farmers graze their animals on a rotation that keeps the growth cycle of the grass revved and running at optimum performance. Instead of dumping their animals' droppings into toxic manure lagoons like the large CAFO operators do, small farmers view their animals' dung as a valuable link in the cycle of life. They compost it and use it to nourish the fruits, vegetables, grains, and grasses that, in their turn, feed the animals and humans.

Small-scale local farms also do more to safeguard a region's biodiversity than large-scale operations. Instead of clearing hundreds of acres of farmland to grow a single crop or raise a single type of livestock, small farmers often produce a colorful menagerie of fruits, vegetables, and animals. It's not uncommon for one farm of less than forty acres to offer more than a dozen different foods. For many small-scale producers, this strategy is smarter than

Your Body, the Dirt in Your Garden: What Do They Have in Common?

I asked Molly C. Haviland, director of the Living Soil Compost Lab, what readers needed to understand about soil fertility in order to make environmentally responsible food choices. She explained that humans and soil share a common biology, and what keeps us healthy is the same process that keeps soil healthy:

Ask any successful gardener their secret to growing delicious, beautiful produce, and they'll tell you it's the soil. Healthy, living soil is key to abundant life on our planet. The soil food web includes countless species of organisms that are macroscopic—seen with the naked eye—and microscopic.

A diverse soil food web offers numerous benefits. First, it's loaded with all the minerals and nutrients a plant needs. These nutrients are released out of the digestive systems of the organisms in the precise form plants require to thrive. Second, the soil naturally retains these nutrients. Billions of organisms create excellent soil structure that won't blow or wash away. This structure allows plant roots to go deep into the ground and permits water to percolate down and be retained.

Third, it promotes disease resistance, because nourished plants have stronger immune systems: they're better equipped to ward off pathogens and disease-causing pests. Fourth, many members of the soil food web break down toxins and pollutants, giving degraded and polluted land a fresh start. And finally, diversity of soil life is essential to a robust ecosystem that will be able to withstand a rapidly changing climate.

Over the past eighty years, extractive farming practices have damaged the soil food web. Excessive tilling breaks up the fungal network that is the circulatory system of the soil and disturbs the soil structure.

Salt-based fertilizers and synthetic nutrients salinize the land and dehydrate the soil.

Classic university agriculture courses tend to focus on "feeding" plants through the addition of nutrients and minerals. This works, but it takes significant energy to mine minerals and create fertilizers. The fact is that Mother Nature has developed her own system for doing this. Just think: billions upon billions of bugs that want nothing more than to eat, reproduce, and poop, twenty-four hours a day, seven days a week. We don't even have to pay them. All we have to do is understand how to be good stewards to them.

So, what can we do to safeguard the soil food web? Organic agriculture is a great start, but it's *restorative* agriculture that's essential to a truly sustainable growing system. If you want to create a compost pile or worm bin, great! You'll see for yourself the way these critters break down organic matter and turn it into black gold. Avoid anything with a name ending in "icide": these chemicals wreak havoc on the little guys, decimating the diversity of beneficial organisms that keep the disease-causing organisms in balance. If you wouldn't bathe in it or hose your kids down with it, why would you put it on something you consume?

Recent studies from the Human Microbiome Project have confirmed that 90 percent of the cells in our bodies are microbial. We are walking ecosystems. Beneficial soil organisms are like you and me. How would you feel if you were put in a sealed bag or if someone ran a tiller through the middle of your house? We are biology; living soil is biology. The complex diversity that makes us healthy is part of the same system that keeps our soil thriving. In recognizing our kinship to the soil, we'll better understand how to nurture the diversity of life.

monoculturing because it safeguards against crop loss. If the peaches don't do well this year, you have the cucumbers, squash, and lettuce. If the chickens have a rough year, the turkeys may offset the loss.

Another way small producers protect a region's biodiversity is by working *with* the terrain, instead of against it. Small-scale farmers often keep some of their acreage in trees because doing this conserves water and provides shade. They step back, look at their land, and let its contours and microhabitats dictate how they utilize their acreage. They may leave a certain amount of it undisturbed so that they can coexist with wild species.

Then, too, small independent farmers can protect the biodiversity of their land because they are able to work in ways that build soil fertility instead of depleting it. Many avoid applying chemicals that kill soil bacteria. They keep the complex microcosm of organisms in their soil alive and active throughout the winter by planting cover crops. They feed it organic material in the form of rich compost. They rotate crops and animals frequently so that harmful pathogens can't get a foot in the door and micronutrients don't become depleted. They look to nature itself for their methods, where life is symbiotic and nothing is wasted.

Food That Doesn't Cause Animals a Lifetime of Suffering

Many people who switch to a local diet do so because they care about the welfare of the animals whose milk, meat, and eggs they consume. They've read about concentrated animal feeding operations (CAFOs), the standard means of production in the industrial food system, and they know that the animals raised this way often suffer unspeakably. The people who switch to local food for this reason have a strong sense of duty toward living things and they feel that we humans have a responsibility to the animals that provide our sustenance. These people want to see for themselves the conditions in which these animals are raised. It's the only way to know for sure that they're being treated well.

Whereas small producers frequently welcome visitors, the CAFO system generally does not. They have an array of policies and procedures in place that keep customers from seeing exactly how their animals are raised, slaughtered, and processed. In these corporate-controlled giant operations, animals are treated as commodities. Their needs, fear, and pain are of no importance. If you've ever driven near a CAFO, your nose tells you pretty much everything you need to know about the lives of the animals inside. The high, windowless walls of the structures in which they're kept tell you the rest of the story. You're not meant to see what's going on in there.

Your local farmer, by contrast, is likely to be proud of the way she raises her livestock and eager to show how it's done. She will demonstrate the great lengths her farm goes to in order to assure that their animals live according to their natures. Their cattle spend their days munching on grass, not agricultural waste. Their pigs root around in forests instead of chewing each other's tails in frustration. Their chickens, whose beaks are never clipped, scratch the dirt for tasty bugs. The animals on these farms are happy, healthy, and respected.

One of my sons' friends argued against this concern for the welfare of animals raised for slaughter. "We're just going to kill them anyway," the kid claimed, "What's crueler than that?" I suspect that people who think this way have not yet discovered that not all slaughtering techniques are the same. An animal can wait hours or days, deprived of food and water, sometimes in an injured or maimed condition, before dying an agonizing death at the slaughterhouse. Or they can be taken right up to the moment of slaughter with a minimum of fear and discomfort.

Some small-scale farmers will actually let you come and watch the slaughtering process. A few might even let you do it yourself, if you're so inclined. They believe that it's good for you to be deeply involved in the procurement of your meat. Far from callous about the death they're dealing, many farmers think that the most honest way to eat meat is to look the animal in the eye and acknowledge it as a living thing before you take its life. It's a more realistic encounter than the supermarket experience, where the sterile rectangle of pinky-red stuff on its Styrofoam tray bears no resemblance whatsoever to the warm, breathing creature it once was.

Food That's Less Likely to Harm the Eater's Health

These days, reading the news is enough to drive a person to seek alternative food sources. In recent years, the American public has encountered dozens of stories about outbreaks of food-borne illness. They've likely heard about the four modern-day super-bacteria that are quickly evolving to outsmart our attempts to control them: E. coli 0157h7, listeria, salmonella, and campylobacter. They've been frightened by stories of tainted meat that's recalled, but not retrieved from stores, and ends up being eaten by unsuspecting consumers.

I was astonished to learn just how many recalls have been issued in recent years because of listeria, salmonella, and E. coli. According to the USDA, in 2010, twenty-six recalls were issued for meat products tainted with one of these three deadly bacteria. In 2011, there were thirty-three bacteria-related recalls. The USDA's public records go back as far as 1994. In each year since, they have recorded numerous recalls of meat products due to contamination by one of these three microbes.

Campylobacter, which comes to us primarily from chicken meat, is quickly catching up to the other three in terms of its fear factor. According to the Centers for Disease Control and Prevention, it's one of the most common causes of diarrheal illnesses, sickening as many as 1.3 million people each year. In 2009, a *Consumer Reports* study found salmonella and campylobacter in more than two-thirds of the store-bought broiler chickens they tested.

Meat gets the most attention when it comes to food-borne illness, but in recent years, vegetables too have had their dark days. In 2011, and again in 2012, lettuce from California tested positive for salmonella. In Oregon in 2011, strawberries tainted with E. coli sickened dozens. In 2012, Kentucky-grown cantaloupes, tainted with salmonella, killed two people and sickened hundreds more across twenty states. In 2013, an outbreak of illness in Arizona was linked to listeria found in broccoli.

This is just a small sampling of the many food recalls that have been featured in the news in recent years. According to the CDC, approximately 48 million Americans get sick from food-borne illnesses every year. That's one in six. Of these, 128,000 are sick enough to be hospitalized, and 3,000 die.

Small local food producers look, to many consumers, like a safer alternative for two reasons. First, if an outbreak is linked to a local farm that only serves its own community, recovering the tainted product will be a far easier task, because the food would not have gone as far. Try recovering contaminated food that is shipped to dozens of states and could potentially end up on thousands of grocery store shelves.

Second, small producers can grow their food and raise their animals using methods that discourage disease. Instead of leaving their cattle, poultry, and pigs standing around in their own filth, they can lodge them on fresh pasture or in airy barns. Because their animals live comparatively stress-free lives and are typically bred and raised for robust health instead of rapid growth, they exhibit less disease, even without the routine inputs of antibiotics that CAFO animals receive. They are also likely to be slaughtered in small abattoirs that process their carcasses at a slow enough rate to avoid contaminating the meat with fecal matter.

This doesn't mean we can assume all foods from the industrial system are roiling with disease, or that all foods from small local producers are safe. Small farms sometimes do have to deal with outbreaks, and labels such as "organic" and "free range" aren't guarantees against disease. Still, for the reasons I've mentioned, many people have come to think of food from small local producers as a safer bet.

Food That Isn't a Product

One exercise we do in my anthropology class involves dividing students into groups of four, giving each group a common grocery store item, and asking them to count the ingredients and come up with a ratio of food to non-food items. What happens next is inevitable: A student raises her hand and asks, "What do you mean by *food?*"

Why do I have to explain to them what food is?

I usually just answer this question by saying it's food if it's something you could grow in your backyard, if your grandparents would have recognized it as edible, or if it has some nutritional benefit to offer you. It's the stuff that, when you read its name, you can picture what it looked like when it was alive and growing. For instance, I can visualize spinach and kale growing green in their soil. I can't do that with maltodextrin, citric acid, or sucralose.

It's worse than you think. It appears that most of them have never read a food label before. If they had, they wouldn't react the way they do.

I'm a really mean teacher. I give them classic college-student favorites such as ramen noodles, mac 'n' cheese, diet cola, and energy drinks. As they go through this exercise, their eyebrows rise higher and higher. "Oh my God," they moan, "I *loved* this stuff!" Now that they've discovered what's in it, they often swear they're never eating it again!

It's not fair for me to pick on my students more than anyone else, though, because, as a nation, we're all pretty food-illiterate. We've gotten so accustomed to processed grocery store items that we've become unable to distinguish *food* from *products*.

Let's make a few things clear. Food is a plant, animal, fungus, or other life form that gives nourishment to humans. Most products are objects designed, produced, and sold for the purpose of making a profit. Nature makes food; humans make products. Food is an edible substance from a once-living thing. Products that are designed to be eaten may *contain* substances that were *manufactured* from food.

Both food and products can be found at the grocery store, but only one of these substances exists in nature. Nobody finds *products* quietly springing up from the forest floor while they're out for a stroll. Nobody grows *products* in their backyard.

A processed edible product can never occupy the same space—nutritionally, economically, ecologically, or morally—as *food*. Let's take for a moment your average energy bar, which plenty of folks think of as a health food. So as not to pick on any particular corporation, we'll make up a fictional one. Let's call it the all-natural caramel mocha Boogie Bar.

Let's compare our made-up product to an egg.

We'll start by looking at their sources. The energy bar came out of a factory production line. The egg came out of a chicken. The Boogie Corporation, which makes the bar, formulates its recipe according to the recommendations of a panel of nutritionists who draw their knowledge from a few decades of accumulated scientific data about the nutritional requirements of a human. The chicken formulates the nutritional content of her egg based on 150 million years' worth of evolution—the approximate length of time the class of egg-laying chordates known as *aves*, or birds, have existed.

The chicken doesn't pack all that nutrition into her eggs for our benefit, but for the nourishment of her offspring. We just hijacked it. Somewhere in our evolutionary history, *homo sapiens* discovered that robbing birds' nests yielded a high-energy snack. We have it backward. Nature didn't whip up a nutritional formula for us and put it in an egg. We evolved bodies that made use of the nutrition available in our environments. Our ancestors developed the bodies we have today on a hunter-gatherer diet, which featured a broad spectrum of seasonal local plant and animal foods, which involved the egg, but never, until the past few years, included the Boogie Bar. Nutritionists surely know a thing or two about human nutritional requirements, but no item assembled in a lab can match the nutritional complexity of foods that evolved over millions of years, as members of an intricate, thriving ecosystem.

Now let's compare the two items from an economic perspective. The egg was created to sustain life. The Boogie Bar was created *to make money*. The energy bar, its recipe, and its logo are patented, because the company has to protect its investment. Can you imagine someone trying to patent an egg? From an economic standpoint, comparing eggs with energy bars is like comparing my Aunt Leona with Donald Trump. If you're looking to get rich, invest in the Boogie Bar. If you're looking to gain the greatest nutritional benefit for the smallest outlay of capital, go for the egg.

How about from an environmental perspective: which one creates the smallest ecological footprint? Making Boogie Bars requires complex machinery and some form of energy to power it. An egg can be made with no machinery at all, other than the biological kind that Mother Nature gave the chicken. Its packaging is all natural, too. You can toss an eggshell straight onto your compost heap. Try that with the Boogie Bar wrapper and you are *littering*.

The egg is also the clear winner when it comes to conserving fossil fuels. You can't make the energy bar in your home. You have to get it from a store, which got it from a warehouse, which got it from a factory. The energy bar may have traveled hundreds of miles before it ends up in your hands. Delivery trucks have to run on something, and honey, it ain't Boogie Bars. By contrast, the egg could have come from as close as your own backyard. If you've got your own flock of glossy, lovingly named hens out back, you don't have to burn any gasoline at all to collect their eggs.

If you can't have your own backyard menagerie, you could get your eggs from a nearby farm. You exchange around $3.50 and some pleasant conversation for a dozen fresh eggs, and you may even exchange a glance with the actual hen that laid them. It's a relationship with a little substance. In contrast, you're not likely to get invited to the Boogie Bar factory, and acquiring one of their products does not entail a relationship of any kind, beyond the thirty-second act of handing over your money to a stranger behind a cash register.

The idea of relationships, and the compassion that they imply, points us to the ethical portion of the argument. If the Boogie Bar was invented to make money, then the only people who can derive sustenance from it are *those who have money*. For the billions of people worldwide who subsist on two dollars per day or less, eating a patented, processed product is simply not an option. But if they have chickens, which are efficient scavengers and recyclers, they can get eggs for no cost.

As a source of sustenance, the egg will always be more available, to more people, more cheaply and efficiently, than the Boogie Bar. We will keep more people fed, and make the world a more equitable place, if we keep in mind that the ideal food for human beings comes from nature, not corporations.

That's the difference between eating *products* and eating *food*.

Food That Nourishes

The people who seek out organic and locally grown food often do so not only to avoid pesticides and reduce their carbon footprint, but because they believe it's more nutritious than what they'd find at the grocery store. They believe that when fruits and vegetables are grown in vibrant soils, when livestock and poultry are raised on the food that nature designed them to eat, and when meat animals are allowed to mature slowly instead of being rushed through the growing process, they develop far denser nutrition.

The people who cite nutrition as a reason for their choice believe that pastured eggs have more omega-3 fatty acids than eggs from hens in battery cages, because they are able to derive more of it from a natural diet of grass and bugs. They believe milk and meat from pastured cattle is lower in saturated fat and cholesterol, not only because of a leaner diet but because foraging animals develop more muscle tone.

Are they right?

Dr. Mehmet Oz, of advertiser-supported radio and television fame, in a December 3, 2012, *Time* magazine article, argued that consumers need not worry about the minimal difference in nutrition between the "farmers' market bounty" and the "humble brick" of frozen spinach they might find in their grocer's freezer. The Mayo Clinic states that a review of articles on organic food and nutrition published during the past fifty years shows that data are inconclusive. Its website, www.mayoclinic.org, advises consumers to assume that organic and nonorganic foods are "comparable in their nutrient content."

In 2008, however, researchers at the Organic Center and Washington State University released a survey of ninety-seven published studies comparing the nutritional content of organic with nonorganic food. Their article showed that organic foods are on average 25 percent denser in nutrients and contain higher levels of eight key nutrients.

Why the contradiction? Is organic food more nutritious or not?

The problem here is partly that we're asking the wrong question, and comparing the wrong variables.

Part of the confusion occurs when people use the word "organic" as a catch-all, assuming that as long as it bears this label, the food in question has all the traits they're seeking. A food item can bear the label Certified USDA Organic and still have been grown by the same large-scale, input-intensive

But Don't I Need Citrus Fruits for Vitamin C?

You might be tempted to argue that you have to break the hundred-miles-or-less rule when it comes to citrus fruits because, after all, most Americans don't live in citrus-growing regions, and how else would you get your daily dose of vitamin C?

According to the National Institutes of Health, men need 90 mg of C per day, and women need 75. The average orange contains about 70 mg of C. That's a lot. But a green pepper contains 95 mg, more C than you need in a day. A cup of strawberries has 83 mg. Tomatoes, spinach, blueberries, and many other non-tropical foods pack a pretty good load of C as well. So even if you don't live in a semitropical region where citrus grows well, as long as you eat a lot of local fresh fruits and vegetables every day, odds are good you're getting your C.

But if you really love oranges, tangerines, and their kin, couldn't you treat them as an exception to the local food rule? If, most of the time, you eat locally the things that can be grown near you, couldn't you just allow yourself some citrus as an indulgence?

monoculture techniques as nonorganic foods. It simply means that artificial chemical inputs (fertilizers, pesticides, and herbicides, mostly) were not applied to the land for three years prior to harvest.

This was the reason food journalist Michael Pollan, in *The Omnivore's Dilemma*, coined the term "industrial organic" to recognize that, even with the most odious chemical inputs removed, food could still be produced using industrial methods such as heavy mechanization, monoculture, and long distribution chains. In fact, many of the organic fruits and vegetables, packaged items, and processed foods sold in supermarkets and large organic chain stores are produced this way.

When I posed the question of nutrition to organic farmer Nick Maravell, he replied, "it all depends on how the food is raised." He explained that what really makes the difference in the nutritional density of produce is the health of the soil in which it was grown. "The food with the highest nutrient content comes from active, vibrant, alive soil." Organic produce grown in depleted soil isn't likely to be more nutritious than its conventionally grown counterpart, but a farmer who uses techniques that focus on soil health grows food with far more nutritional density.

Nick claims that this is especially true when it comes to animal products. It's the animals' access to pasture that makes the greatest nutritional difference. On grass, he explains, "animals are exhibiting their natural behaviors and are in contact with the soil. It's how they live in nature." Nick explains that it's this healthy soil, and eating the grass grown on it, that allows the products of pastured animals to be higher in omega-3 fatty acids. He feels that the more time animals spend in contact with soil, the better, which is why his cattle never go inside.

Some of the farmers I've spoken to suggest that there's one foolproof way to test the nutritional content of the food you buy: *listen to your body*.

I learned this trick many years ago. My friend Sarah, from my college years, was a die-hard health food freak. She taught me that the true test of the healthfulness of the foods I ate was in the way they made me feel. Does a particular food give me long-lasting, clean-burning energy, and a clearer mind? Or does it leave me feeling muzzy, sluggish, and run down? When I apply the Sarah Test to the foods I'm eating now, the answer is clear. I feel much better when I eat fresh, whole food from local sources.

My whole family concurs. Since we've been eating this way, we've had fewer illnesses of any kind. We've slept better. We've laughed more. We've had the energy to exercise more often. Granted, we're just one family. That means our results make for anecdotal evidence at best. By all means, conduct your own research. Try eating local foods for a month and then check in with yourself. How do *you* feel?

Food That Is Honestly Priced

The number one argument I have heard consumers give *against* local food is its higher cost: "Why would I pay five dollars for a dozen eggs when I can get them at the grocery store for $1.99?" They automatically assume that the lower price they pay for the CAFO eggs is the fair price. That leads them to conclude that the higher price for the organic pasture-raised eggs is *unfair*, and that any farmer charging that much for her eggs is greedy.

Let's look at the real reasons for this price difference. First, it would be a mistake to assume that small-scale farmers are asking a higher price for *exactly the same product*. A pasture-raised chicken, egg, or beef cow is not at all the same thing as a chicken, egg, or cow from a CAFO. An organic, vine-ripened heirloom tomato might as well be a different *species* from the mass-produced grocery store tomato. You get what you pay for.

For the past century, large-scale food producers have focused primarily on high yield and low cost, rather than on quality. The result is that the food from supermarkets and restaurants often leaves us unsatisfied and disappointed. Because they operate according to a different set of goals, small-scale independent growers simply produce better food. As we'll discuss in Chapter 12, one consequence of the higher quality is that it takes less of it to satisfy you, so you tend to eat smaller portions. That alone could help offset some of the higher cost.

Finally, small producers have to charge more per unit for their food because government policy, as it's currently written, makes production more expensive for small operations. In many ways, the federal government rewards large businesses and hinders small ones.

When you take all these issues into consideration, you can view local food's sticker shock in a different light. It's the price you pay for grocery store food that is unrealistic, whereas the price charged by your local farmer is more likely to reflect the true cost of production.

Throughout this book, I'll show you how to make a few adjustments so that you and your family can enjoy great local food for less than your current grocery budget, even though the upfront cost for many of the items you'll purchase will be higher.

Food That Makes an Abundant Living for the People Who Grow It

Speaking of profit, when you spend that $151 to $180 each week to feed your family—according to a 2012 Gallup poll, the average national cost for a family of four—who do you think should benefit from that money? Do you want most of it to go to the farmer who grew the food, or to the chief executive officer of the corporation with whom the farmer has a contract?

Americans spend billions of dollars per year on food. Somebody is getting stinkin' rich, and it's not the guys picking the strawberries. The Bureau of Labor Statistics estimated the mean wage for farm workers in 2012 at $29,570. Meanwhile, the online news outlet *Arkansas Business* reported that Tyson Foods' CEO Donnie Smith made $7.8 million in 2012. The *Chicago Tribune* reported that Kraft Foods' CEO Tony Vernon brought in $9.19 million in 2013. According to the *Omaha World Herald,* ConAgra Foods' CEO Gary Rodkin's total 2013 compensation clocked in at $10.7 million. Who are you really supporting with your food dollars?

By contrast, small-scale farmers often feel a sense of duty toward the farmhands who work for them. One of my noncredit students, a man who had been farming for several decades, told me that he went to great lengths to pay his hired help well, year-round, even though doing so ate deeply into his profits. He sold firewood culled from his forested acres during the winter months, not because he could make a profit from it, but so that he could keep giving his farm workers a paycheck during the off-season.

If we think about it, we want our farmers and their helpers to be paid well. These are the people who grow the stuff that keeps us alive. We want them to have an incentive to keep on doing it, and to do it the best that they can. In the corporate world, the name of the game is "maximize profit." To the typical small farmer, the ultimate goals are to "keep people fed and employed" and "care for the land." He may never get rich doing this, but as long as we give him our business, he can make a comfortable living at it.

Food That is Available to All

We live in a world where food is not equally available to all people. This year, approximately 870 million people worldwide will not get enough to eat. Yet, here in the United States, we stuff so much extra food into ourselves that, according to the Centers for Disease Control and Prevention, 69 percent of us are overweight and 35.9 percent are obese.

For the struggling populations of the world, the best hedge against starvation is to ensure that they have access to a living wage and the ability to own and control the means of making a living. The reasons any given group of people can't do this range from economic inequality to political instability, and in many parts of the world, communities are facing a very long road to a future in which they will be able to feed themselves securely.

But how does my decision to eat local food in Maryland help my hungry neighbor in Haiti, Ethiopia, or Bangladesh? Just because we'd like to see struggling populations feed themselves securely and independently, from sources that strengthen their local economies, why does that mean we have to do the same here in the U.S.?

I think it has something to do with practicing what we preach.

Solving a problem of this magnitude involves, among other things, cultivating the right attitude. If we're serious about food equality, then we have to be ready to live it. If I dine sumptuously on imported caviar and sixteen-ounce steaks every night, something that most people on this planet *cannot* do, it won't have an immediate, quantifiable effect on any starving person in the world. But it has an effect on me. It has an effect on my place in the world, as I understand it.

I'm not saying we all have to live an ascetic lifestyle. I much prefer the idea of everyone living abundantly. But eating mostly simple, local food that was produced with a minimal footprint is just one more way to position ourselves on the road to a more egalitarian world.

Another way to approach this subject is to say that we want the human food supply to remain under the control of *people*, rather than corporations or political entities.

All populations deserve to have the same access to the global food supply that Americans have. But alongside this kind of food security, it would be a good idea for all of us to cultivate a certain amount of food security closer to home.

Does the President Eat Local?

Believe it or not, since 1800, every sitting president of the United States has had access to ultra-local food, produced right on the White House grounds. Not only home to several vegetable gardens, including the one installed in 2009 by First Lady Michelle Obama, 1600 Pennsylvania Avenue also maintains its own beehive and brewery. The honey from the commander-in-chief's bees is used to craft the signature presidential brew, White House Honey Ale.

No one in the world needs to go hungry for want of seeds to plant. Whenever I cut into a pepper, a pumpkin, or a tomato, I'm overwhelmed by the sheer number of seeds inside them. You can grow a wondrous variety of vegetables yourself just by removing the seeds from the ones you bought at the farmers' market, then planting them next spring. I know this is true because 100 percent of the potatoes, pumpkins, butternut squash, acorn squash, and garlic that grew in my garden last year was obtained this way. Farmers of centuries past saved the best seeds from each year's crop for planting next year. They never even needed a seed catalog, let alone a patented product from an agricultural lab.

Knock on your neighbor's door in mid August and ask for some of the seeds from their zucchini; you'll go home with more than you know what to do with. Knock on the door of a giant agribusiness research and development lab and ask for some of their patented seeds; call me from your cell at the police station and let me know how it went.

Do I sound like a conspiracy theorist when I say this? Does it seem a bit out of sync with the present reality of twenty-first century America to say that we should be fervently scraping the seeds out of our cantaloupes?

At the present, we in the United States have an abundant and super-reliable food supply. But pull the lens of history back to a wider focus for a second. Recall the victory gardens of World War II, the Dust Bowl of the 1930s, and the Civil War. In those times, in many parts of the country, food supply lines were cut. Are we so confident that we will never again face a long-term disruption to our food supply that we want to abdicate all of our agrarian knowledge?

Food security in the modern world is defined as access to a global food supply. We could add to this definition of food security by also defining it as a state in which sufficient tools, materials, farming knowledge, and access to land reside within the community itself: in the hands of the people. Food security defined this way is not dependent on any business entity, government structure, or institution. It needs no charitable handout. It endures so long as the community itself endures.

Food That Enhances Connections

One of the reasons people express dissatisfaction with our current economic system is that it has caused a certain amount of estrangement between us and the items we buy. We have almost nothing to do with the

GMOs: Genetically Modified Organisms

A genetically modified organism (GMO) is produced by directly manipulating an organism's genome. It's typically done in an attempt to give the organism a desirable trait. For instance, scientists have created a GM tomato that contains DNA from an Arctic flounder, in the hope that the tomato will be as cold-resistant as the fish. It sounds like science fiction, but this technology has already been integrated into the American food system, mostly without our knowledge.

You have probably eaten quite a few GMOs, whether you were aware of it or not. Although the overall percentage of your food that has been genetically modified is probably small, GMOs have become quietly ubiquitous in the American diet. According to an October 2012 *USA Today* article, approximately 88 percent of our feed corn and 94 percent of soybeans are genetically modified.

The use of GMOs raises several concerns. First, the insertion of foreign genes into an organism doesn't take into account the fact that any species' genes are integrated and work together in a highly complex interrelationship. Since gene splicing is an imprecise procedure, its overall effect may not come to light for many generations.

Second, consumers who have merely asked that they be informed about which of their foods contain GMOs have found that some of the companies who produce foods with GMOs are refusing to identify them as such. Some GMO food manufacturers have even fought food producers who don't use GMOs and simply wish to label their products as "non GMO."

Third, GMOs can be patented by their developers, which may set a legal precedent for the ownership of life forms and the concentration of food sources in the hands of big business. This mind-set runs against the idea that access to food, because it's necessary for sustaining life, is a fundamental right of all people, not a tool for concentrating wealth in the hands of the few.

Finally, GMOs encourage an input-intensive model of farming. Organic farmer Nick Maravell explains that the use of GM crops begs the use of pesticides: "GMOs were introduced to be pesticide-resistant. If you don't use pesticides, there's no reason to use the GMOs." He notes that GMOs, first developed more than thirty years ago, have already been a common part of the agriculture industry for almost two decades, and they have yet to show the miraculous results originally promised. "If GMOs were a silver bullet, we'd have seen it by now." In spite of this new technology, farmers still deal with crop loss. "It's just another tool that a farmer has," Nick explains. "In this case, it's a question of how useful that tool is." According to Nick, the use of GMOs may have added to the problem: certain weeds, now called "superweeds," have become resistant to the pesticides used with GM crops.

There's much around the issue of GMOs that calls for an honest, open, respectful dialogue. I've heard an awful lot of mean talk around GMOs and few attempts from either side to reach out and understand one another. I wish that the pro-GMO folks would respectfully agree that it is not hysterical or paranoid to raise concerns and ask questions, nor is it unreasonable to ask to be informed about what is in one's food, nor does it make a person anti-technology to question the effects of a particular technology. I wish that the anti-GMO folks would remain open to the notion that scientific research and innovation may very well have the potential to solve *some* human problems, and that we'll never fully know what any new technology may do unless we give it a try.

origins of the stuff we consume. We have little to no idea how, or where, or by whom it was produced, and when we're done with it, we throw it away, without another thought to what happens to it after we dispose of it. We have little to no bond with the people who make the stuff we consume or the people who sell it to us. Our hollow transactions have cultivated an ignorance in us that we can no longer afford.

Many of us are casting about for a better system.

Food is the best place to start rebuilding those connections, because it's so fundamental to our survival. When we buy local food, we end up participating far more deeply in its story. Every head of lettuce has a history. It was germinated from seed somewhere, it grew in a particular patch of soil, and it was exposed to its region's weather. At least one pair of hands tended it on its way from field to market. Now it has passed from that person's hands to yours. You complete the story when you take that once-living thing into your body and incorporate it into your own being.

Because it requires a deeper level of involvement, local food draws us into a meaningful interaction with nature. Eating locally involves visiting farms, catching our food in the act of growing, knowing what grows well in our region, and discovering what's in season. It goes a long way to reteaching the agrarian wisdom our culture has lost, to reconnecting us with the rhythms of Earth.

Buying local food also helps to strengthen community ties. The local food movement is part of a bigger socioeconomic trend toward local commerce. Nationwide, many Americans are looking to regain the sense of connection to their neighbors that they had decades ago. They feel that the sterile, fleeting, stranger-to-stranger interactions at the cash registers of giant national chain stores just aren't a very honorable way for humans to interact. They see value in ongoing relationships, the kind that are made when economic transactions happen between neighbors who have more at stake in their interactions than their bottom line.

The local food movement tends to lead to stronger connections with family and friends, too. This kind of food doesn't come to our tables without effort. We have to prepare it—an activity best shared with loved ones. Unlike the fast food slurp-and-go type of eating that's usually done solo in the car while you're on the way to something else, real meals are not conducive to multitasking. They're to be savored, enjoyed along with the company of those sitting down to eat with us. They bring you fully into the moment.

Food That Tastes Amazing

Oh, and there's one more thing I need to tell you about local food: this stuff tastes *incredible!* It satisfies like no fast food burger has *ever* done, even in its wildest dreams.

Please, don't just read about this experience in a book. Go visit your local farm and taste the difference for yourself!

What Local Food Is Not

Just to be absolutely clear, let me also tell you a little bit about what local food is not. Some people come to the local food movement with expectations that it isn't going to meet. Let's head these off at the pass.

Local food is not snob fare. It's not fancy gourmet provender for discerning diners. If you look at what's on offer at most farmers' markets, CSAs, and farm stores, it's humble grub: turnips and collard greens, not capers and caviar. Eating local is not a thing you do to improve your social image. It has more to do with your view of yourself than anyone else's opinion of you.

Local food is definitely not a miracle weight loss plan. There's a reason you haven't read about the Local Food Diet in the news. I believe it's a much healthier way to eat, but will it make you skinny in less than six weeks? Don't count on it. It's not a cure for obesity, although it might help, depending on what local food you eat, and how much. If you fry your sustainably grown chicken in organic lard, and finish off your meal with three scoops of ice cream from pastured dairy cows, you'll be just as fat as you would have been if you'd eaten the same foods from the grocery store.

Local food is also not a fix for anybody who's hooked on convenience. If you aren't willing to invest some of your time, energy, and creativity to eat this way, it's probably not going to work for you. There's more to this movement than just buying the same old stuff, only locally. It's a sea change, a paradigm shift. It requires a change in lifestyle. You will be investing more of yourself in the part of your existence that has to do with eating. Instead of just cramming the most readily available stuff into your mouth whenever you're hungry, you'll be cultivating a food life.

On a similar note, local food is definitely not about having it your way. A value has crept into our culture that is patently destructive and wasteful, and it's known as instant gratification. It's the mind-set of "happiness is having

The Top Ten Local-Organic-Sustainable Foods That Taste Way Better Than Their Supermarket Equivalents

1. Fresh local organic tomatoes
2. Milk from grass-fed cows
3. Eggs from pastured hens
4. Pasture-raised chicken
5. Ground beef from grass-fed cows
6. Fresh organic local cheese from grass-fed cows or goats
7. Organic pasture-raised pork
8. Fresh local organic cucumbers
9. Fresh local organic peaches
10. Fresh local organic sweet corn

How to Choose a Farmer

Mary Kathryn Barnet of Open Book Farm in Myersville, Md., offers this advice for families who are looking for a farmer: "Think about what's most important to you. What are the qualities you're looking for in the food you're eating? Is it the specific growing method, the cost, or animal welfare?"

Although their farm is not certified organic, the Barnets raise both organic and nonorganic chickens, so that their customers have a choice. The organic chickens cost a dollar more per pound because that's the additional cost they incur when they raise birds on organic feed.

If you're not sure what method your farmer uses, or if you have any questions about the way your food is raised, you can call up the farmer and ask. "People should always feel that they have a right to ask polite questions," M. K. explains. "You should be able to know what you're getting."

whatever I want the instant I want it." That's not freedom; that's addiction. Fast food restaurants feed this compulsion. So do supermarkets that offer thousands of choices. This attitude isn't making us into nobler creatures.

By comparison, eating local food is about making choices within the limitations set by nature. When you commit to eating most of your food from local sources, you become conscious of the fact that food has seasons. You learn that the best time to eat a given food is when its harvest time comes, and during the rest of the year, you eat something else. You rediscover the sweet, aching pleasure of anticipation, and the rapture of enjoying a food whose time has finally come. You learn to discipline your cravings. You discover that desires that are cultivated and channeled, when they're finally satisfied, bring the most intense bliss of all.

Local ... Compared With What?

So, when we talk about local food, with what are we comparing it? The antonym of local food, as we're discussing it here, isn't just food that comes from far away. It's food that was produced in the industrial system.

This is the food production system that habitually uses monoculture, CAFOs, large-scale production, artificial fertilizers, pesticides, herbicides, pharmaceuticals, and enormous amounts of machinery, infrastructure, and fossil fuel. It's the factory method of agriculture that treats living things as parts on an assembly line and demands that they be uniform. It's the system that defines efficiency as fastest, cheapest, and highest yield, rather than most sustainable, most nutritious, or most equitably available. It treats food as a commodity to be bought and sold, not as a necessity for sustaining life. It's governed by the corporate goal of maximizing profit, rather than the humanitarian goal of meeting needs. It's run on a closed-door, need-to-know policy that fosters consumer ignorance rather than consumer empowerment.

Industrial agriculture and processed foods are at the far end of the continuum from what we're calling local foods because they do next to nothing to strengthen the physical, emotional, or economic health of communities aside from supplying calories. In the name of short-term efficiency, the industrial food system wastes energy transporting items that could have been produced closer to their point of sale. It produces with little regard to the sovereignty of living things or the health of ecosystems. It spends millions

Industrial Food vs Local Food

INDUSTRIAL	LOCAL
Large scale	Small scale
Mostly corporate	Mostly family owned
Focus: corporate profit	Focus: civic responsibility
Goal: maximize profit	Goal: serve community, care for the land
Government subsidies	Fewer government subsidies
Mostly commodities	Mostly produce
Long distribution chain	Often farm to consumer
Advertising	Mostly word of mouth, reputation
Closed to public	Transparency of method
Monoculture	Many are diversified
CAFOs	Some are free-range, cage-free
Chemical inputs	Some are organic
Hormones/antibiotics	Some are hormone-/antibiotic-free
Extractive	Some focus on building soil health
Heavy fuel consumption	Minimal fuel consumption
Heavy infrastructure	Lighter infrastructure
Ship nationally	Ship shorter distances
Packaged	Little or no packaging
Artificial inputs	Some focus on natural, on-site inputs
GMOs	Some are GMO-free
Small number of varieties	Some focus on biodiversity
Food science	Environmental stewardship
Grown mostly for processing	Mostly for fresh consumption
"Extreme" flavor	Natural flavors
Year-round availability	Seasonality
Shelf life	Freshness
Vitamins added	Soil complexity = nutritional complexity
Convenience	Requires time and energy
Strangers	Neighbors

on advertising and public image, but it has been known to actively fight regulations that would inform its consumers.

Fortunately, if we decide we don't want to eat food that was produced this way, we have options. Our response to this system doesn't need to be a rebellion, a boycott, or a court battle—nothing that rude. We're simply choosing to get some, if not most, of our nourishment from a different source. We're not trying to run anybody out of business. We're not seeking to shut down the industrial food system. We're simply opting out.

You'll Never Eat a Total Stranger

So this, in a nutshell, is what local food is, and what it's all about. These are the reasons people are opting into a lifestyle that centers on fresh, whole, locally grown produce.

This movement is not an isolated phenomenon, but part of a much larger picture. It's the beginning of a shift in human consciousness, an awareness of the awesome power we have to shape the fate of our world. We have it within our means to be the most destructive force Earth has ever known, or to be the nurturing shepherds of our planet. It's a choice that's incumbent on each of us.

Within our lifetimes, we'll have few opportunities to make a huge impact on the world, but we have a chance to make a little impact several times a day. Over a lifetime, all of those small-but-lovingly-made choices add up. We have an opportunity to exercise this choice every time we decide what's for breakfast, lunch, and dinner. Instead of chowing down thoughtlessly on whatever's convenient, we can make our meals an act of *intimacy*.

This is the soul of the local food movement: consumption as a fully conscious act, eating with eyes wide open.

Rocket Fuel Red Slaw

My husband, Al, and I devised this recipe after finding an entire, very intimidating, head of red cabbage in our CSA bag. This slaw can be made with 100 percent fresh local ingredients during their growing seasons.

2 cups roughly shredded red cabbage

1 roughly shredded carrot

1 small sliced onion

4 cloves minced garlic

1/2 cup mayonnaise

1 tablespoon white vinegar

1 teaspoon dill

1 teaspoon dried hot red pepper seeds

Shred the vegetables in big chunks, so they stay toothsome and crunchy. Combine vegetables in a large bowl. Combine mayo, vinegar, dill, and pepper seeds in a small bowl. Pour mayo mix over vegetables and stir thoroughly. Chill, then serve. Note: this stuff is awesome in sandwiches!

4

How Did We Come to Prefer a Twinkie Over a Tomato?

A Brief History of Human Eating

When a man moves away from nature, his heart becomes hard. —*Lakota Proverb*

My kids were fifteen years old the first time they tasted Twinkies. About a year ago, they had a rare opportunity to try some of these iconic crème-filled treats, not because I had bought them, but because a student had brought several boxes of them to the final class of the semester as a gag, since I had made an example of the ubiquitous Twinkie during a lecture on economic systems. She had passed them out to the class, and then insisted that I take the leftovers home to my boys.

As they chewed, I asked them what they thought.

"Ridiculously sweet," was Phillip's assessment.

"Like eating a pillow," said Ben.

My sons are probably a statistical anomaly. Plenty of kids would dine on Twinkies for breakfast, lunch, and dinner if they had their druthers. What determines why one kid turns up his nose at a particular food item, while another one eagerly chows down?

Human food preferences are uniquely complex. Our tastes are driven not just by caloric needs, but by history, culture, genetics, associative memory, values, habits, and a host of other intangibles. Like other social animals, we humans feed ourselves collectively. The decisions about what, when, with whom, and how much to eat are made by the group, rather than the individual.

You may argue that you made the decision to have that peanut butter and jelly sandwich for lunch today all on your own, but you didn't. The bread on which you smeared your peanut butter came to reside in your refrigerator as a result of an incalculable number of decisions, ranging from the U.S. government's policies that subsidize grain production, to European colonists' choice to bring this particular grain to the new world in the 1600s, and all the way back to our Middle Eastern predecessors' decision to domesticate wheat's wild ancestor more than eleven thousand years ago.

Because food choice is never as simple as it appears, we'll need to take a holistic view of our society's relationship with food to understand why so many modern Americans have come to view a Twinkie as desirable.

How Food Shapes Society

Food is so basic to our survival that the means by which we get it carves the contours of our entire society. If you tell an anthropologist how a particular community obtains its food, she can predict the approximate size of the group, the kind of religious system they have, what motivates them to work, their marriage practices, family structure, the way they govern themselves, and maybe even the sounds of their music and the look of their artwork.

Just to throw in a little bit of perspective, I'd like to introduce you to a few of the *other* ways human beings have fed themselves, and the shaping effect these systems have had on their societies. Without these other food-getting systems for comparison, we might be tempted to think that ours is the only, or best, or default way of getting people fed. But when you look across all cultures—all people, all places, all times—you find you're looking at a very different picture.

Hunter-gatherers. Hunting and gathering—foraging for wild plants and animals—was the only means of making a living for the first two million years of our existence. It predates our species by around a million years and was the exclusive way of life for all human beings for 97 percent of the time we've been on Earth. It built the bodies and the psyches we have today and, according to some nutritionists, it's the way we should *still* be eating: lean meats, fish, leaves, roots, nuts, berries, and few grains.

Hunter-gatherers grew no crops and domesticated no animals, other than (eventually) dogs. They foraged everything they needed from wild sources. They lived in small, nomadic, kin-based bands, governed by the informal leadership of elders. They were communal—they shared whatever they had—and egalitarian—they didn't divide people into classes or castes. Status between men and women was often closer to equal here than in many other kinds of societies. People in hunter-gatherer bands worked, not for cash, but to fulfill social obligations. Throughout their lifetimes, they worked alongside the same people with whom they lived and played.

Few groups still live as hunter-gatherers today, and many have lost their traditional foraging territories to agriculturalists. Some still do it part-time,

No Wonder We're Not Getting It

On Friday, January 17, 2014, on the 5:00 a.m. news, our local TV station ran a story with this lead: "Fast food may have little to do with obesity." You bet that got my attention!

The story cited a recent study by the University of North Carolina at Chapel Hill that found that the habits that lead a child to develop obesity start early in life, with unhealthy foods served in the home. The reporter concluded that this combination proved to be far more of a factor in obesity "than the child occasionally eating fast food."

The study, led by Barry Popkin, professor of nutrition, indicated that the majority of obese children were regularly eating too many fatty foods and sugary beverages both at home and at school. In other words, it's not that fast food has little to do with obesity, it's that, by itself, it's not the only culprit in an overall pattern of unhealthy food choices.

But that's not the headline they ran for this story. The conclusion they drew from the UNC study was that fast food has *little to do with obesity*.

On Monday, February 3, less than three weeks after they ran that headline, the same news station ran a story on their midday news with this lead: "Fast food *does* have a fast effect on the body." They cited the work of U.S. and Irish researchers that indicated that fast food "increases the average BMI 0.03 percent per serving."

BMI, or body mass index, a ratio of mass to height, is used to indicate whether an individual is overweight or obese. A person is considered overweight with a BMI of 25, and obese with a BMI of 30 or more.

According to the British online news outlet *Daily Mail*, this new claim is actually an interpretation of research published in the World Health Organization bulletin that linked the rise in the number of fast food meals consumed to the rise in average BMI. Between 1999 and 2008, the average number of fast food meals eaten per year per person rose from 27 to 33, and the average BMI rose from 25.8 to 26.4.

Around the same time as these findings, a study was released by the University of East Anglia drawing a direct correlation between childhood obesity and the proximity of fast food restaurants. The closer kids lived to these places, the higher their rates of obesity. Likewise with the number of such establishments in their neighborhoods: the more fast food restaurants nearby, the higher the obesity rates among kids. The rates were higher for middle-schoolers and older kids, probably because they had more freedom and pocket money.

Coincidence?

as a way of preserving their heritage. Our current generation may see the extinction of this way of life. Could we all go back to living as hunter-gatherers? Not a chance. Although this way of life makes a much lighter impact on the environment, it can only feed a tiny, sparse population. Earth couldn't possibly support seven billion hunter-gatherers.

Horticulture. Horticulturalists grow and raise most of their own food in small, temporary garden plots. Their farming techniques are simple, and most of the work is done by hand. Horticulturalists are seminomadic. They farm an area for as long as it stays fertile, usually between three and five years. Each family farms its parcel until the fertility is tapped out. Then the whole village picks up, moves to a new spot, and starts the whole process over again, letting nature reclaim the previous plot.

Horticulturalists can still be found in various parts of the world today, although they too are finding themselves pushed off their lands by large-scale commercial agriculture. Women typically do a lot of the work in these societies, so polygyny—one husband with many wives—is common. More wives equals more hands to do the work of feeding the family.

Horticultural societies are typically larger and more complex than hunter-gatherers', but they too are aware that their lifestyle has limits. They typically plant crops that don't store well, such as bananas and yams, and they seldom have access to refrigeration, so they don't really have the option to put aside a little extra in order to trade up to a lusher standard of living. In fact, many horticultural societies have cultural restrictions on excess. For instance, among certain traditional societies in New Guinea, when pigs got too numerous and started flattening people's kids and rooting up the gardens, villagers planned a massive pig fest. They invited neighboring villages over, slaughtered all those extra pigs, had a massive barbeque, and sent everyone home happy.

Pastoralism. The pastoral way of life centers on raising herd animals. Reindeer are essential to the Sami of Finland, as camels and goats are to the Tuareg of North Africa, and cattle to the Maasai of Kenya and Tanzania. Pastoralists typically graze their animals on land that's too scrubby and barren for most other subsistence activities to be practical. Even where crops can't grow well, grass can often thrive, and although humans can't eat grass, we can graze our animals on it and then eat the animals.

A Duty to Share: The Way of Ningiqtuq

The Gwich'in, an Athabaskan hunter-gatherer group in eastern Alaska and northwest Canada, believe that everyone's entitled to food and shelter. The Gwich'in word *ningiqtuq* conveys the sentiment that individuals, families, and communities have a duty to share what they have with those in need.

Historically, pastoralists have made an easy and abundant living. There's not a lot of work to do, and food is readily available. Children often have important roles to play in pastoral societies, as milkers and guardians of the herds.

You'd think that, if herd animals are the centerpiece of a pastoralist's life, then steak would be on the menu most nights. But one of the features of pastoralism is that, even with loads of animals to eat, they typically prefer to leave their herds alive, which makes a certain economic sense. You don't slaughter your wealth unless you have to, or unless it's quite a special occasion. A dead cow gives you meat for a few days. A live one can provide milk; blood; dung for cooking fuel, roofing and flooring material (you can do a lot of exciting things with manure); and new baby cows.

Agriculture. An agricultural way of life is very different from the three I've mentioned so far. Where hunter-gatherers, horticulturalists, and pastoralists live a nomadic or seminomadic existence, agriculturalists keep large expanses of land under permanent cultivation. This system can grow an enormous amount of food and feed large groups of people, and it can do so reliably, most of the time. When it does fail, the results are catastrophic, because a large, settled population can't move as readily as a smaller one. Agriculture usually makes a greater impact on an ecosystem than foraging, horticulture, or pastoralism, because it permanently alters the landscape and reduces the biodiversity of a region.

Agriculture produces so much food that it allows a small percentage of the population to feed everyone else, freeing the majority of the people to specialize in other kinds of work, such as pottery, metalsmithing, or writing books about local food. It's the only way we've devised so far to feed a large, dense population, such as a city, so it's the only form of subsistence that can support what we call civilization. Agriculturalists typically use complex techniques and machinery, and they require a well-organized labor force, and thus demand a different kind of social structure. In these societies, a centralized government maintains control over the workforce, and it can enforce its will on the people because it can support a judicial system, police force, and standing army.

When you compare agriculture-based societies to any of the more traditional systems, the first thing you notice is the social stratification. Life in a society that relies on intensive agriculture is typically marked by the greatest extremes of wealth and poverty. With a population this large and dense,

Bet You Never Felt This Way About Your Cheeseburger

To the Maasai, pastoralists of Kenya and Tanzania, cattle are wealth in and of themselves. The Maasai name each cow and sing songs about their herds. To many Maasai, eating the flesh of cattle is an activity infused with meaning, connecting them to their heritage. Although the Maasai have been under pressure from the Kenyan and Tanzanian governments to abandon their traditional way of life, the humanitarian aid group Oxfam International has praised their system of seminomadic grazing as a relatively sustainable way of making a living in the face of climate change.

most people are strangers to each other and therefore an economic system governed only by social obligations doesn't work here. Instead of reciprocity, an exchange of goods or services in the context of a relationship, civilizations rely much more on commercial exchanges—in other words, money.

Industrial Agriculture. After covering hunter-gatherers, horticulturalists, pastoralists, and agriculturalists, most anthropology textbooks stop. But there's a fifth subsistence system, different enough from the other four to warrant its own category: *industrial* agriculture. This is the system that has risen to dominate the American food system in the past five decades, and the one that is rapidly spreading across the globe.

The hallmark of this form of production is large-scale monoculture: stripping an area of hundreds of native species in order to grow a single domestic species as a commodity and as quickly, cheaply, and in the largest quantities possible.

The industrial agriculture system may have begun as a means to offset the high costs and low profit margins of small-scale farming, but it has risen to power in a contemporary economic climate that favors large-scale business models over small. It seeks to maximize the profits derived from food production by streamlining production methods, creating the largest possible quantities as quickly as possible, and minimizing the cost of production.

Industrial agriculture makes a mighty profit for the shareholders and CEOs of large corporations. It does little to provide an abundant living to farm workers and food service employees.

It is, of course, the most efficient food production system invented, so long as you define "efficient" as "lots, fast, cheap." If your definition of efficiency includes any ideas such as "environmentally responsible," "economically equitable," or "great tasting," industrial agriculture does not deliver.

Yet, to most contemporary American taste buds, industrially manufactured foods have become the norm.

A Brief History of Human Eating

We all have a hunter-gatherer somewhere in our ancestry. Until about twelve thousand years ago, it was the only way of life we knew.

Our great-great-great-granddaddy, *homo erectus*, invented this way of life when he got the bright idea to use stone tools in a new way: not just to chop

When the Soil's Compromised, It's Game Over

The Hohokam, ancient farmers of Arizona whom we know only by archaeological record, prospered long enough to build more than 150 miles of irrigation canals. Yet, by 1400 A.D., their society had mysteriously vanished. Evidence suggests that their way of life collapsed because soil salinization gradually poisoned their farmland.

High Tech = High Inequality?

Although it has created wealth and a higher standard of living for many, the price of industrialization has been high. Industrial societies are characterized by high rates of inequality and heavy impacts on their environments.

11,500 years ago
First agriculture

780,000 years ago
First *Homo sapiens*

1.8 million years ago
First hunter-gatherers:
Homo erectus

Subsistence Timeline

We humans were exclusively hunter-gatherers for more than 97 percent of our time on Earth.

off scavenged meat from the kills of other predators, but to do a little hunting of his own, strategically coordinating his efforts with his buddies. Many paleoanthropologists claim that cooperative hunting, and the organized social relationships it demanded, launched our ancestors on a trend toward larger and larger brains. It also caused them to migrate. They left Africa and followed the herds into the Middle East, Europe, and Asia, adapting their way of life to each new environment as they went. This was the way of life for all humans until about twelve thousand years ago.

So what changed? If hunting and gathering had gotten the job done for all that time, why did prehistoric humans begin growing their own food? What was the motivation? I've asked students to speculate on this question, just to see where their assumptions take them. Here are some of my favorite *wrong* answers:

"They finally got smart enough to figure out how to plant their own food." Nope. Our ancestors' brains reached modern-day cranial capacity around 780,000 years ago. They weren't lacking in the brains department. Besides, hunter-gatherers typically possessed an intimate knowledge of plants. They knew how to make them grow if they chose to. But why go to all that effort as long as all the food you need is growing wild right outside your door?

"They got tired of working so hard." No, farming is much harder work than foraging. Hunter-gatherers typically worked fewer hours per day than we agriculturalists do.

"They finally had the technology to invent agriculture." Actually, the first agriculture used relatively simple tools. Agriculture eventually produced enough surplus to feed labor specialists, who were then able to develop complex technology. First came the farming, *then* came the technology, not the other way around.

"They were motivated by a desire to progress." The students who say this might be imagining a bunch of Neanderthals sitting around a bare cave on a dripping wet evening with nothing to do. "You know, there's gotta be more to life than this. Let's invent the karaoke machine." Progress is mostly a modern value. In a society where it's possible to amass surplus and become wealthy, where status is associated more with personal gain than with personal relationships, it makes sense to want to progress.

According to geological, climatological, and archaeological records, our ancestors' decision to become farmers seems to have been motivated by two factors: population growth and a climate shift. For the majority of the time our species has existed, people were thriving on a hunter-gatherer lifestyle and gradually populating the globe. Eventually, the population of hunter-gatherers reached critical mass. Groups began to bump into each other, and to elbow each other out in competition for the best foraging grounds.

Also at this time, the world experienced a radical shift in climate. At the end of the Pleistocene, the last big ice age, the climate became unstable and plunged into a series of wild fluctuations.

For both these reasons, humans at this time began to cast around for other ways to feed themselves. Groups that were pushed into marginal environments began to try to recreate the abundance they remembered from their previous territories. At first, they simply did what any good hunter-gatherer knows how to do in lean times: they saved back some seeds and gave wild plant species a helping hand.

Every season that they did this, they selected seeds from the plants that had the traits they liked best. Year after year, they bred the plants that were hardiest, most flavorful, or easiest to harvest. Over time, they began to change the DNA of the species they were cultivating. What they were doing was called *domestication*. The domesticated crops and herds we have today are as different from their wild counterparts as a Boston terrier is from a gray wolf.

Domestication began first with plants around twelve thousand years ago. Herd animals were added to the mix later. This crop-animal-human collaboration was mutually beneficial for everyone involved. Humans could harvest their crops, and turn their animals out to graze the remains, guarding them against predator attacks. The animals, as they ate, would fertilize the soil for next year's crop. They also provided a steady supply of meat, milk, and hides.

Among the earliest farmers, certain groups were geographically blessed. Anyone who had access to cereal grain, such as wheat, barley, rice, or corn, had an advantage: they could feed a much larger population. This was especially true for those groups that also had access to great herd animals, such as sheep, goats, cows, and pigs, and most especially if they had an animal that could pull a plow.

This is why civilization sprang up around the Fertile Crescent in the Middle East and developed almost everywhere the people of the Middle East migrated, including into Europe, and eventually, into the Americas. The whole process went a bit slower in the New World because, although they did have corn, amaranth, and llamas, a llama is too slight of build to pull a plow.

In his book *Guns, Germs, and Steel*, Jared Diamond explains that the

Eskimo Science: You've Got to Be Smart to Make It as a Hunter-Gatherer

Ethnographer Richard Nelson studied the Kuyokon, a group who live just below the Arctic Circle in Alaska's interior. He describes them as some of the most uniquely adapted people in the world. As with most hunter-gatherers, the encyclopedic knowledge they carry—about plants, animals, terrain, weather patterns, seasons, and natural cycles—could fill many scientific volumes. Over a lifetime, the Kuyokon strive to learn, not only *about* animals, but *from* animals, because, as an elder once told Nelson, "each animal knows more than you do."

farmers in the parts of the world that didn't have these advantages couldn't support as large a population and couldn't feed any of the specialists—metalworkers, potters, anthropology teachers—that keep a civilization thriving. Over time, many areas that didn't have naturally occurring grains and herd animals acquired them as imports. But even in modern times, nations and peoples who didn't fare as well in the "geographic lottery" are still struggling to compete with those that had a head start.

Many of the agricultural societies that had access to high-yield cereal grasses and multipurpose livestock animals flourished and gave rise to states and nations as we know them today. But farming, for all its benefits, led humanity into something of a vicious cycle. Every time humans invented a new food-growing technique, the population grew, requiring still more innovations.

Where most Westerners have been taught to view civilization as an unequivocal positive, anthropologists tend to think of it as a mixed bag. The rise of civilization has enabled arts, sciences, technologies, discoveries, and a remarkable synergy of knowledge and understanding. But it has also brought inequality, poverty, malnutrition, famine, epidemics, and environmental collapses. It has put humans at the top of the list of destructive forces that are changing the face of our planet.

How Food Production Became Big Business

Although any form of agriculture has the potential to damage its environment, throughout this chapter, I've differentiated industrial agriculture from other forms. The earliest agriculture was practiced, not to generate profit in a cash market, but to sustain the lives of a populace. *Industrial* agriculture is practiced, first and foremost, to generate a profit.

Money, as we know it, is much younger than farming. Agriculture existed for more than six thousand years before the first form of monetary exchange. Heavy metal ingots, the precursors to coins, were first used as a form of exchange in Mesopotamia around five thousand years ago. Crops grown for their commercial value followed shortly thereafter.

During the European Colonial Era, five hundred years ago, an increase in the demand for raw trade goods spurred the development of faster, cheaper means of turning raw items into finished products. Cities became central hubs of production. This trend toward urbanization and mechanization lay the groundwork for the Industrial Revolution, beginning about three hundred years ago. This era saw the rise of coal-fired machinery and factory assembly lines, and it led to the birth of the "fast, plenty, cheap" notion of efficiency.

The Industrial Revolution triggered massive change in American society. Throughout the nineteenth century, we evolved from a rural, agricultural society to an industrialized, urban nation.

It was the beginning of the end of a way of life that had stood the test of time for millennia. The culture that grew out of the Industrial Revolution became part of our daily lives. To this day, we educate our kids in neat little rows of desks, in a one-size-fits-all configuration inspired by the efficiency of the assembly line. This mind-set also laid the groundwork for the rise of industrial agriculture.

How Green Was the Green Revolution?

In the two decades after World War II, biologist and humanitarian Norman Borlaug spearheaded a series of initiatives aimed at increasing food production worldwide to meet the demands of a growing population. The Green Revolution, as it came to be known, brought about a massive increase in the use of high-yield and hybridized crops, irrigation techniques, pesticides, herbicides, and monoculturing, and greatly increased the production of certain types of foods worldwide.

In the decades since its inception, the world has seen a decline in severe poverty and famine. Yet, this movement has come under harsh criticism for the means by which it brought about this apparent salvation. It has been denounced as environmentally disastrous and unsustainable. The monoculture techniques it favors require the application of large amounts of pesticides, and the high-yield varieties it promotes require large inputs of fertilizer. Monoculturing itself reduces a region's biodiversity by growing a small number of varieties over large areas.

Today, the term "green" is often used synonymously with "environmentally sustainable." In this terminology, the admittedly life-saving Green Revolution was anything but green.

Others have criticized the movement for bringing unequal benefits. While many parts of the developing world vastly increased their yields, the Green Revolution initiatives didn't have as dramatic an effect in African countries. Still others have made a case that, historically, where famine has been rampant, the cause can seldom be chalked up to lack of agricultural techniques, but rather to a combination of socioeconomic problems, government corruption or repression, and political unrest.

A major influence in the global shift to industrial agriculture, the Green Revolution remains a controversial and hotly contested movement. Did the Green Revolution save millions of lives? Almost certainly. Could those lives have been saved by using a different strategy—one that favored long-term environmental sustainability and economic equality? That's the answer we're really looking for.

The colossal food industry is one aspect of a trend toward bigger and bigger business in our society. Just as giant banks, colossal media companies, and massive telecommunications firms have busily devoured their competitors, large food companies have been buying up smaller ones. It's become harder for small-scale businesses of all kinds to stand firm in the shadows of giants.

How Food Tastes to Humans

If you're like most modern Americans, you've become accustomed to the highly orchestrated flavors in processed foods. If you've never tasted anything else, then this sensory input is normal for you. But what you're tasting when you bite into a chicken nugget, corn chip, or microwave meal, is not the flavor of *food*, but a carefully manipulated sensation that is the result of laboratory research and chemical alchemy.

All food manufacturers are aware that the more mechanical processes a food item goes through, the less of its natural flavor it retains. This goes even more so for any food that's designed to sit on a grocery store shelf for months at a time. The result is that, in order for these foods to taste like *anything*, food manufacturers have to add artificial flavorings to compensate for the fact that the real flavor is long gone.

Did you ever read the ingredient label on a food item and wonder what the phrase "natural and artificial flavors" referred to? They are nearly the same thing. These are any flavors or aromas, derived from extracts and chemical compounds, added to foods and beverages. Without them, that microwave pizza would taste about the same as the cardboard box it came in.

But food manufacturers don't add artificial flavor concoctions just to restore lost flavor. They have the science of taste down to an art form. According to Eric Schlosser's *Fast Food Nation*, some of the larger food companies employ scientists whose goal is not just to make the food taste acceptable, but to make it taste so outrageous, so extreme, and so addictively delicious, that you'll sell your grandmother just to get your hands on more of their product.

It's not so much the "natural and artificial flavors" in processed foods that are the problem. It's three other ingredients that combine with these flavor compounds to produce an orgy of sensations on our taste buds. According to Michael Moss, in his book *Salt, Sugar, Fat*, processed foods would be all but

Choose My Subsidized Plate?

Remember the old Food Pyramid from the 1980s? Nah, neither do I.

In 2011, the USDA revised its recommendations for daily nutrition and published it in the form of the Choose My Plate campaign. Their new graphic features a dinner plate divided into four sections labeled fruits, vegetables, grains, and protein, with a separate circle, apparently representing a glass, labeled dairy.

But when the question of nutrition is posed to the Physicians Committee for Responsible Medicine (PCRM), they respond with a different set of guidelines. Citing the mounting body of evidence that shows a link between animal products and obesity, hypertension, heart attack, stroke, diabetes, heart disease, coronary artery disease, and certain types of cancers, they've created the Power Plate, which features four equal portions of fruits, legumes, grains, and vegetables. No meat, no eggs, no milk.

The USDA does mention nuts and legumes as a protein choice, and in the dairy category, it offers the option of soy milk. But meat, poultry, seafood, and eggs top its list of proteins, and all its other dairy choices are animal-based. The PCRM suggests vegetable-based proteins only, and it leaves out the dairy category entirely.

Why would these two plates be at odds? Why would the USDA encourage us to eat up to a third of our calories per day from sources that the PCRM claims are damaging to our health?

Could the USDA's plate be a compromise between the foods that are good for us and the industries that command the largest number of food subsidies? Sixty-three percent of the U.S. food subsidy budget goes to meat and dairy, 20 percent to grains, and less than 1 percent to fruits and vegetables. If we ate our meals proportionate to the way the government subsidizes them, meat, dairy, and grains would dominate the plate, and the fruits and vegetables we'd consume would be the size of one skinny string bean.

I don't know why this mismatch exists. But I do know that the USDA is tasked with the dual mission of supporting public nutrition *and* promoting American agriculture, which includes the beef, pork, poultry, and dairy industries. What can we expect it to do when those two agendas are at odds?

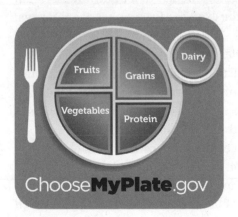

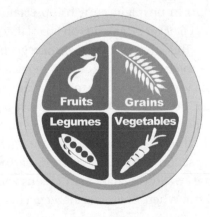

The USDA's Choose My Plate program, left, recommends dairy products at every meal, along with vegetables, fruits, grains, and proteins. The Physicians Committee for Responsible Medicine recommends the Power Plate, right: an equal balance of fruits, vegetables, grains, and legumes—no meat, no dairy.

inedible without the addition of those three substances, any one of which, in a large enough quantity, can be lethal to a human being.

All three of these substances are necessary to our survival. To our hunter-gatherer ancestors, fatty, salty, and sweet foods were rare delicacies. Fatty meats and ripe, sweet fruits meant dense calories, which spelled survival to a people perpetually on the move in search of their next meal. Natural selection has hardwired us to love the taste of fat and sweet. Our bodies reward us for ingesting these things.

Sodium chloride (aka salt) amplifies other flavors, so food tastes bland without it. In tiny quantities, it is necessary for proper metabolic function, and it has been especially important to human survival as a food preservative. It also seems to have a certain addictive quality: the more you add, the more accustomed you become to large amounts of it in your food. And processed foods are generally oversalted to maximize flavor.

The marvelous thing about the human taste apparatus is that, because it can be conditioned, it can also be *reconditioned*. If you're a salt addict—as I was and, to an extent, still am—you're not doomed. You can gradually reduce your salt intake to a reasonable level, until foods that barely seemed salty to you before taste almost unbearably briny. Likewise with sugar: sweetness is on the tongue of the beholder. My kids found a Twinkie mouth-puckeringly sweet because they're used to eating foods with little or no added sugar.

The experience that waits for us outside the world of artificially devised flavorings is the fact that *real food* has *real taste!* Compared to the neon-bright blasts of added chemical flavorings, the genuine flavors that nature builds into food are subtle, complex, and endless in variety.

If you're a skeptic, what's probably going through your mind now is, "Yeah, a grown-up might learn to appreciate the exquisite flavor notes of a rutabaga, but I'll never get my kids on board that train. Kids naturally despise vegetables."

This is a myth. The taste of vegetables is not inherently repugnant to kids. It's the form in which those veggies usually appear on their dinner plates. The vegetables most American kids consume come from a frozen block or a can. Freezing and canning remove a great deal of a veggie's fresh flavor and impart a few flavors that rate high on the "yuck" scale.

If you're close to my age, you might even recall a certain spinach-chomping sailor, of Saturday morning cartoon fame, who pushed the propaganda that swallowing dark leafy greens will make rock-hard pecs burst from your chest. Where did this seafarer get his spinach? Not from his backyard garden or the farmers' market, but out of a can! Only canned vegetables require this kind of PR. Fresh spinach doesn't need a burly sailor as its spokesman.

The sad fact is that many, perhaps most, American kids today are unaccustomed to the taste of truly fresh fruits and vegetables. When fresh food is what is normal to them, most kids eat their vegetables happily. This goes doubly so if the vegetables and fruits they're eating are ones they've helped to grow, or helped to select from a farmers' market stand. In my household, fresh spinach, steamed and lightly buttered, is one of the most popular side dishes. There are never any leftovers.

Food preferences are mostly a matter of familiarity. Cheese puffs taste normal to kids only because someone has encouraged them to eat them on a regular basis, and to view them as an appropriate food choice.

What Food Means to Humans

Human taste is driven by familiarity, and the matter of which foods are familiar to us is dictated by our culture. No human society eats every edible substance within its environment. Everyone has a set of cultural prescriptions about what's good to eat.

Some cultural food prescriptions are driven by environmental circumstances. I once had a student who told the class that he had frequently eaten dog meat in his home country as a child. The people in his village didn't have the option of driving to the supermarket to pick up a package of ground beef any time they were hungry, and his elders raised him with the idea that meat from any source provides valuable protein. The class reacted with disgust to his story, because Americans tend to view dogs as companions, not lunch. The student confessed that what disgusted *him*, when he first came to this country, was our habit of eating cheese: "You wait until your milk is so rancid, it's solidified, and then you *eat it?*" He said it had taken him years to get up the courage to try a cheeseburger.

I'm fascinated by food customs, especially those surrounding the world's grossest foods. Whenever I have a student who hails from Scandinavia, I have to ask: have you ever eaten lutefisk? This traditional Swedish dish literally translates to "lye fish," which is exactly how it's made. Aged whitefish carcasses jellified in a caustic solution. This stuff is so pungent that, legend has it, it once grounded an aircraft. Apparently, a man was carrying a jar of it in his on-board luggage. When the jar broke, the putrid odor drove everyone off the plane. Yet many students tell me with pride that they eat lutefisk every Christmas. It's a matter of tradition, maybe with a dash of machismo. Your ability to ingest geriatric seafood dissolved in lye marks you as a true Scandinavian.

Humans, alone among all other living things on the planet, eat food not only for its taste, but for its meaning. Food manufacturers understand this, which is why they develop whole ad campaigns around the meanings their products deliver and the emotional states they promise.

As twenty-first century Americans, it's become part of our cultural programming to seek extreme experiences. It's the best way for retailers to ensure that we keep on buying: never let the customer remain satisfied with what she's already tried.

Burst of flavor! Extreme cheesiness! Outrageous fruitiness! These phrases shout at us from processed food packages. They have to yell in bold lettering because they're competing with dozens of other food products for our grocery dollars. They've got to have an advantage over their competition in the flavor department because they know they'll lose the nutrition argument. Outrageous taste is all they have to hook us with.

Time to Stop Eating With Our Eyes Closed

Fortunately for us, we have an opportunity to learn from our past. We're now coming to understand that the price of eating well is constant vigilance. We can't trust the processed food industry to give us products that are truly in our best interest. We can't rely on a government agency with a split agenda to advise us about our eating habits.

What do we do, going forward? This is a matter of individual decision. One person might feel drawn to government activism; another might take on corporate misbehavior in a court of law. Another course of action—a quieter, gentler, but no less powerful one—comes in the form of the decisions we make as consumers. Although the industrial food system has made it a point to be ubiquitous, we can still make different choices.

Culture is changed in precisely this way: when a significant part of the society sees a need to adopt a new way of doing things, especially when that new way resonates with their lifestyle. Even though we've been encouraged to believe it, we don't have to accept that a Twinkie belongs in the same mental category as a tomato.

Choosing Whole, Fresh, Local Foods for Optimal Health

What's the connection between the so-called diseases of affluence and the typical American diet? What is it about the foods we're eating that's fueling this disastrous trend toward obesity and the host of diseases that follow it?

Recently, I posed these questions to Dr. Louise Stomierowski, a family practice and emergency medicine physician with thirty-five years of medical experience, who also revealed to me that she had struggled with weight issues throughout her own life. She told me, "There is no doubt that our modern dietary intake and sedentary lifestyle directly affect our risk of developing hypertension, diabetes, endometrial cancer, prostate cancer, colon cancer, and stroke."

But what is it, *specifically*, about the American diet that's problematic? According to Dr. Stomierowski, It's the high levels of fat and empty carbs in the foods that are the cheapest and most abundant in our society: "All the food we eat is turned into glucose, the only sugar our body cells can burn. Carbohydrates such as breads and cereals, and proteins such as meat, eggs, and beans each release four calories per gram. Fats, any foods that leave a grease stain, have the greatest density. Each gram yields nine calories." The carbs in candy, cake, and soda provide almost no nutrients, only empty calories our bodies convert into energy so quickly that large amounts can throw our metabolism into hyperdrive. "The immediate increase in blood glucose triggers stress-related digestive patterns in the body, and these extra calories are stored as fat in the body if not offset by activity needs."

But if eating this way is so damaging to our health, why do so many of us do it? According to Dr. Stomierowski, "As we have been blessed with an extraordinary choice of foods and activity levels, we have been cursed with the opportunity to make poor selections." She cited many reasons people make less-than-healthy food choices, including "ignorance, desire for immediate gratification, perceived lack of time, and learned patterns."

She explains that all the up-to-date dietary studies recommend eating fruits, vegetables, whole grains, low-fat dairy products, poultry, fish, nuts, and olive oil to help prevent chronic diseases. The average adult needs six to eight servings of fruits and vegetables a day, which amounts to two cups of fruits and two and a half cups of vegetables a day. As to which fruits and vegetables those are, she recommends, "Buy locally and seasonally whenever possible. Vary the colors." She also emphasizes that eating the right foods is only half of the equation. Great health also requires a moderate level of activity.

I asked her which healthy foods work best for her. She told me she's fond of whole-grain oatmeal: it's cheap, widely available, and has excellent fiber. "I add nuts, raisins, blueberries, cinnamon and skim milk for daily breakfast." She also advocates what she calls "meaningful snacking": making a conscious effort to choose real foods for in-between noshes, such as bananas or popcorn (not the movie-theater kind that's drenched in butter, or "butter").

Dr. Stomierowski validates those of us who struggle to eat right by acknowledging just how difficult it can be. "Trying to find a healthy eating pattern is a lifelong effort," she says. "It's much easier when you're not responsible for preparing meals for others and you have less stress in your life and more regular sleep."

Frying Pan Chili

This is an easy, quick-fixer for busy weeknights. It's flexible—you can throw in whatever you've got on hand—delicious, filling, massively healthy, and takes less than half an hour to whip together.

4 large, very ripe, juicy tomatoes (or a 16-ounce jar of diced tomatoes)

2 large bell peppers

1 large sweet onion

1 medium zucchini

1 small stalk celery

1 cup cooked or canned chili beans

1 block of firm tofu, cubed

1 small Anaheim, jalapeno, or cayenne chili (if you like a little spark)

4 cloves garlic

1/4 cup olive oil

2 tablespoons red curry paste

1 teaspoon cumin seeds

1/2 teaspoon coriander seeds

Mince the garlic, celery, and chili. Cut the other vegetables into large wedges, planks, or chunks. Hang onto the juices, especially the ones from the tomatoes.

Heat the oil in an extra-large frying pan. Add cumin, coriander, garlic, and celery and sauté for about three minutes. Add the beans and the other vegetables and sauté for about ten minutes. Mix the vegetables by turning them with tongs as they cook. Add the tofu and red curry paste and cook for ten more minutes. Serve over rice or pasta.

Part 2

A Practical Guide to Local Food

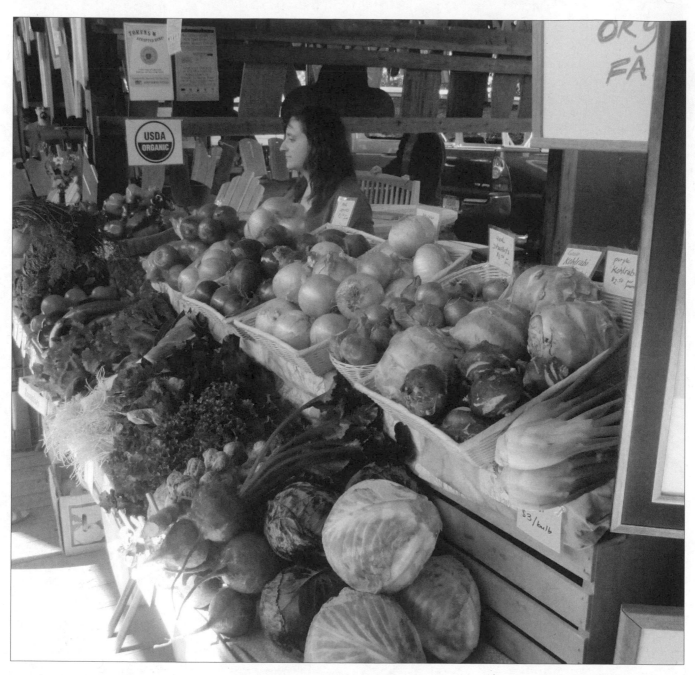

Organic produce for sale at the Ithaca Farmers Market.

5

It's Only Natural

How to Speak the Language of Local Food

A crust eaten in peace is better than a banquet partaken in anxiety. —*Aesop*

Counterculture, flower power, free love: social movements have a way of sprinkling the language with invigorating new words, like a fresh splat of fertilizer onto weary soil. Not surprisingly, this latest era of thinking about food has produced a vibrant new crop of words. Some of these terms are confusing, and worse, misleading. Because I don't want you to end up frustrated, puzzled, or bamboozled by advertisers, I've devoted this next chapter to the lexicon that's forming as people describe the current food landscape.

Why does it matter what words we use to describe food? Anthropology explains that words aren't just inert carriers of meaning; they also influence our thoughts. The symbols with which we describe reality affect our perception of it. Advertisers and public relations firms know this fact all too well and use it to manipulate our opinions of their products. Other people, often with the best of intentions, end up giving the wrong impression of a food production method simply by being a little too vague with their word choices. For these reasons, we need to sort the literal meanings from the connotative.

We'll start off by shining a little light on a few of the trendy words you've probably encountered on food packaging. We'll look at some of the food-growing terms that are good to know if you're developing an interest in the way your food is produced. We'll finish with a quick reframing of the reason why "local" is still the cleanest word to describe the food we're craving.

Is 'Artisanal' the Opposite of 'Industrial'?

Have you eaten anything lately that had the word "artisanal" on its label? I bet it was cheese.

Artisanal cheeses have been enjoying immense popularity of late. The word means made by an artisan, or craftsperson, as opposed to a factory. But what exactly differentiates an "artisanal" cheese from its mass-produced counterpart? According to anthropologist Heather Paxson, many small-scale cheese makers claim their cheeses possess *terroir*, a quality no factory-made cheese could ever have, even in its wildest daydreams.

The French word *terroir*, which Paxson defines as "the taste of place," is the idea that certain foods have a flavor that is distinctive of the region they come from, and it usually refers to wine. Lately, small-scale cheese makers have borrowed this term to differentiate their creations from commodity products.

Paxson writes that terroir, as it's now being used among many small-scale "artisanal" producers, suggests that unique "ecologies of production" create "distinctive sensory qualities in handcrafted agricultural products." Unlike industrial commodity cheese manufacturers, who use unvarying, standardized processes in a sterile environment, American artisanal cheese makers vary their techniques according to seasonal and environmental conditions, with flavor at the forefront of their endeavors. According to Paxson, these cheese makers are harnessing the French vintner's term terroir to help consumers see the value of their ecological stewardship and commitment to their region.

Food Terms: Fluffy, Fair, or Fabulous

You may encounter any of the following terms on food packaging, store signage, or in advertisements. This gallery of words runs the gamut from practically meaningless to spot-on. A few of these terms are trying so hard to mean *everything* that they mean next to nothing at all. Some of them are not entirely devoid of meaning, but are potentially misleading, have definitions that are a little at odds with their common usage, or are otherwise fuzzy around the edges.

All Natural. From a legal standpoint, this term is all but meaningless. It's often used to say that the product contains no chemical *ingredients*, though this doesn't say that the ingredients themselves were produced without chemical inputs. In U.S. labeling, its usage is inconsistent and unregulated. A highly processed product can bear the words "all natural" on its packaging. The Food and Drug Administration has no official definition for this term. Companies deploy this phrase because it makes people assume that the product is wholesome. When I ran an Internet search on it, the search engine returned dozens of porn sites. If this is what the phrase "all natural" conjures in people's minds, no wonder advertisers love it!

Cage Free. Cage free only means that: no cage. Poultry raised this way could still have spent their lives confined in a building, crammed elbow-to-wattle with thousands of their companions. Cage-free birds, like their caged counterparts, often have their beaks burned off. They may be permitted to express some of their natural behaviors, but not all of them. Cage free is significantly better than the "battery cage" system, the standard procedure in industrial agribusiness that crams animals into wire compartments too small for them to stretch a wing or turn around, but it means little beyond this.

Certified Humane. The term "Certified Humane Raised and Handled" is a designation given by the nonprofit organization Human Farm Animal Care to livestock producers who adhere to their strict guidelines regarding the amount of space their animals have, their access to fresh food and water, and the methods used to handle and slaughter them. This group is endorsed by the American Society for the Prevention of Cruelty to Animals and the Humane Society. If a package of meat or a carton of eggs carries this label, it's a sign that regard was given to the animals' welfare.

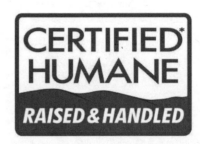

The Certified Humane logo indicates that the animals that produced the product have been treated in accordance with the guidelines set by the Humane Farm Animal Care organization.

Fair Trade. This is the label applied to products sold in the United States that meet international standards for equitable economic exchange, as determined by organizations such as World Fair Trade Organization and Fairtrade International. These standards rate a product's manufacturer according to the ecological soundness of its production methods, the way it treats its labor force, and its economic development practices. The run-together version of this word, "fairtrade," refers specifically to the certification system run by Fairtrade International (FLO). If you're trying to be a local food purist, this term won't enter your lexicon very often, because it's usually seen on imported foods such as coffee, tea, sugar, and chocolate. But if you're okay with allowing yourself a certain number of imported goodies, this label is a very good sign.

Free Range. This term doesn't mean the animals live a vagabond existence on wide-open prairie. It simply means they can move about at will outdoors for at least some of the time. The USDA does regulate the use of this term, requiring water, food, and shelter to be available to "free range" animals.

Grass Fed. When I ask students, "What's the natural food for a cow?" they chime in unison, "Grass!" When I ask them what's fed to most cows in the United States today, their answers range from "corn" and "hay" to "poop." The ones who say this last one think they're being witty, but it turns out they're not entirely wrong. As a cost-saving measure, CAFO cattle are sometimes fed agricultural byproducts that may include, among other things, chicken manure. Yet every schoolchild knows that the natural food for a cow is grass.

Grass is also an essential part of the diets of chickens, turkeys, pigs, sheep, and goats. If "grass fed" or "pastured" appears on a meat label, that's good, but the important question is, how long was the animal's acquaintance with that grass? Did they spend *all* of their lives on pasture, or did they end up in a CAFO for the last six months of it? The phrase that's even more spot-on than "grass fed" is "grass *finished.*" According to the Cattlemen's Beef Board, for beef, this means the animal felt grass under its hooves and dined on pasture for the entirety of its time on Earth.

Green. When you see this term in labeling and advertising, it's appealing to the activist in you. The word is there to make you feel as though you're being environmentally responsible if you buy it. But can you comfortably assume that "green" products are good for the environment?

As of this writing, the American Marketing Association offers guidelines for the use of the term, and the Environmental Protection Agency recognizes standards for "green" products, but there is no specific legal definition for this word. Products that carry the word "green" may or may not make a smaller impact on the world's ecosystems and resources than comparable choices. With each "green" product you buy, you'll have to do a little more investigation to know for sure.

Heirloom/Heritage. These two terms refer to the variety of plant or animal. An heirloom variety is one that's been around a while. It is time-tested and was likely developed to suit the environmental conditions of a specific region. People who grow heirloom and heritage foods swear by their beauty, charm, and exquisite flavors. For instance, the Little Marvel garden peas I'm planting this year were developed in 1908 for their hardiness and sweetness, and they have been the darlings of home gardeners for decades. By definition, a heritage plant is open-pollinating: it can produce fertile seeds with the aid of wind, birds, insects, or other natural means. The fact that it does this leaves it open to genetic variety, so it helps to safeguard biodiversity.

Non-GMO. This phrase on a package label means the food inside contains no genetically modified organisms, meaning no one's invaded the genetic structure of the plant or animal and fiddled with its DNA. Many people harbor grave concerns about food that is genetically modified. Unfortunately, they've probably been eating it for years without realizing it. Although you'll occasionally see products labeled "Non-GMO," I'll bet you a plate of homemade cookies you haven't seen a label that reads "Contains GMOs!"

Aside from the question of whether it's safe to eat them, there's another reason many people give for avoiding GMOs. It has to do with the idea that food is not just a commodity but also a human right. Although a few GM varieties have been developed to boost crop yields in developing parts of the world, most of them were genetically modified for the express purpose of making somebody a whomping big profit. An army of corporate lawyers stands ready to defend their CEOs' right to get rich off of those patented, modified foods. By contrast, we want food to remain accessible to as many people as possible. At a minimum, we'd like to exercise our right to know what's in our food. Bottom line: "Non-GMO" is a good sign, because these products help protect people's right to inform themselves about what they're eating.

Organic. In the United States, the USDA maintains a strict legal standard for foods labeled "Certified Organic." To bear this moniker, food must be, among other requirements, grown without synthetic fertilizers, pesticides, or herbicides, and on land that has been free of these things for at least three years and is routinely inspected.

Achieving Certified USDA Organic status is no simple task. It requires so much paperwork and other time commitments that many small-scale farmers, who typically operate on narrow profit margins, have elected not to pursue Certified USDA Organic certification. The certification for organic farming is extremely lengthy and time consuming. Many farmers follow most of the same methods as Certified USDA Organic farmers, but they've chosen to forgo certification.

"Certified Organic" products have many of the qualities we're seeking in our sustenance, but they're not guaranteed to have them all. Organic alone isn't the whole picture—hence the next term.

Industrial Organic. We've talked in previous chapters about "industrial agriculture," and with all the affection we have for the word "organic," it's tempting to conclude that "organic" is the opposite of "industrial." It's not.

In his book *The Omnivore's Dilemma,* journalist Michael Pollan coined the term "industrial organic" to refer to large-scale food producers who use some of the methods of organic farming, especially the avoidance of antibiotics, hormones, and certain chemical-based fertilizers, pesticides, and herbicides, but who in every other respect could be considered members of the industrial food system.

Many popular organic brands, the kinds you can find in grocery stores across the United States, can be considered industrial because they are mass-produced, different from other grocery store fare primarily in the fact that their chemical inputs are nonsynthetic. How does "industrial organic" square with the kind of food that's featured in this book? Well, it's not the devil. If you're addicted to soy milk, pasta, or breakfast cereal, like we are, there are few local choices, and organic is at least a step in the right direction. But when it comes right down to it, "industrial organic" isn't local food.

Beyond Organic. A good bit of the confusion we're experiencing over the word "organic" results from people thinking that this is all a food needs to be in order to solve the problems we have with our food system. Cutting out the synthetic chemicals does go a long way in the right direction. It helps with certain health concerns and a few of the environmental issues. But it leaves out the facets of this problem that have to do with local economics and social equality. In some cases, small-scale producers end up in a paradox. They can't cover all these bases at the same time, and sometimes have to prioritize one over the other.

In *The Omnivore's Dilemma,* Michael Pollan quoted Virginia farmer Joel Salatin describing his farm as "beyond organic" because, although they don't have an organic certification, Polyface Farms strives for a high degree of sustainability—higher, Salatin asserts, than the "Certified Organic" label reflects. He believes that the overall health of the land and the local economy trump a strict adherence to organic methods.

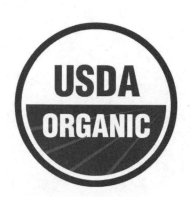

The Certified USDA Organic label indicates that the product bearing it contains 95% or more of organic ingredients.

The term "beyond organic" is also sometimes invoked by farmers who feel that the notion of "organic" has changed a bit since the USDA has involved itself. Some farmers feel that the procedures the USDA requires in order to meet its organic standards cost them so much time, trouble, and expense that they are a distraction from what they consider to be their *real* job: growing high-quality food.

The takeaway point here is that just because a farm you like doesn't carry the "Certified Organic" stamp of approval doesn't mean it can't give you the kind of food you're looking for.

Sustainable. This term, like organic, can mean different things to different people, but the idea behind it is that sustainably grown food doesn't severely deplete or damage the environment in which it's raised. It doesn't shortchange tomorrow's eaters for the sake of feeding today's. What seems to make this a controversial term is that people argue over exactly how sustainable a given practice is, or whether claims of sustainability are accurate.

Some purists believe that a practice should only be called sustainable if it produces at least as many food calories as the sum total of the calories (that is, artificial inputs of energy in any form, including petroleum) it took to raise it. Others—and I fall firmly into this camp—believe that sustainability is relative, and that a move from a highly unsustainable food source to one that's more sustainable is a step in the right direction, especially if we keep on stepping.

Biodynamic agriculture. This method of food production was originally developed by philosopher Rudolf Steiner in the 1920s. It brings a spiritual dimension to organic farming practices and emphasizes the farm as a holistic system of interrelated parts. To a biodynamic farmer, soil, plants, and animals work in harmony to form a unit. Biodynamics also incorporates rituals believed to draw mystical and cosmic forces to enrich the fertility of the land.

That's a lot of verbiage. I'm pretty sure our hunter-gatherer ancestors never had to plow through half a dictionary just to enjoy a good meal. Fortunately, there is an easier way. The surest tactic, if you want to beat the label game, is to eat foods that don't have any labels. One of the most refreshing aspects of buying food directly from your local farmer is that the production methods don't need to be described to you because ... *you're there*. What you see is what you get.

Buzzwords From the Local Food Frontier

What follows next are some agricultural terms you'll bump into when you enter the world of sustainable food. At first glance, you might think these terms are more appropriate for an aspiring farmer in her first year of studies at an agricultural college than for someone who just wants to shop for great local food. But these words, technical though they may sound, are describing some of the basic mechanics of nature. As you ease into the community of food growers and local food eaters, you'll hear words like these to describe how our sustenance is produced.

Biodiversity. The total number of species, and their variations, a community contains. Industrial agriculture and urban development deplete biodiversity. The most sustainable farming practices preserve the biodiversity of an area by growing many different kinds of plants and animals, nurturing soil fertility, and coexisting with wild species.

Diversified. This word means that the farm grows many different kinds of foods. Typically, diversified farms grow both plants and animals, which benefit from one another in a symbiotic system. By doing this, they're helping to preserve biodiversity. It's the polar opposite of monoculture.

Ecosystem. A complex natural system made up of a group of organisms and their habitat. Sustainable farming treats cropland and pasture as ecosystems, and it recognizes that living things exist within a web of interdependency.

Erosion. The wearing away of topsoil as a result of rain, wind, flood, or exposure. This is what all farmers struggle to avoid.

Food Co-op. A food distribution outlet owned by consumers. Food co-ops often focus on healthy, natural, and organic foods, and they have a strong culture of social responsibility.

Food Forest. This is a term from the world of permaculture (see its entry below) that describes an interdependent, multilayered food-growing space that incorporates natural cycles and is designed to enhance, rather than deplete, the ecosystem it belongs to.

Food Hub. A co-op or other business entity that collects, distributes, and markets the produce of a group of local farmers, and may also perform other related services. The USDA defines a food hub as "a centrally located facility with a business management structure facilitating the aggregation, storage, processing, distribution, and/or marketing of locally/regionally produced food products." Food hubs are a growing phenomenon, though many of them

Tuscarora Organic Growers: A Producer's Co-operative Allows Small-Scale Farmers to Work as a Community

In 1988, three organic farmers in south-central Pennsylvania put their heads together to try to solve a common problem: they had little time outside of working their farms and selling at farmers' markets to adequately meet the growing demand for produce from restaurants and food co-ops. Because they worked six days a week on their farms and spent the seventh day at the farmers' market, their primary source of revenue, they decided to hire someone to manage their business relationships with shops and restaurants so that they could concentrate on doing what they did best: growing great food.

As their cooperative took shape, the farmers found that they could also coordinate their choice of produce. With each farmer specializing in the items he grew best, instead of competing, they were better able to serve their customers. Over the years, the cooperative welcomed more farmers and reached out to more customers. Today, TOG is made up of more than forty-six member farms and works with around a dozen more. It delivers more than 120,000 cases of produce annually, and all of the food it sells still comes from sustainably managed small farms. In addition to marketing, sales, and production coordination, TOG also provides its farmer-owners with quality

assurance, based on standards the members agree upon, plus group ordering for growers' supplies.

Recently, I spoke with Tuscarora Organic Growers' Account Manager Jeff Taylor. He explained that, although most of TOG's sales are to restaurants and retailers, about 18 percent of their produce is sold to the farmers themselves, so that they have a wider range of offerings to sell through CSAs and farmers' markets.

I wondered how the local-sustainable food movement looks to folks like TOG who were in the business long before organics were hot. Jeff claims that the popularity of local-sustainable food, although growing, is not new. "The Baltimore-Washington area has always had a local perspective. D.C. and Baltimore have always been accustomed to bringing local stuff in," he explains. "It's been amplified in recent years, but it's always been there." He says TOG plans to continue to ride the wave and quietly grow along with the movement.

The USDA lists Tuscarora Organic Growers on their 2014 Working List of Food Hubs. TOG, and organizations like them, are part of a growing movement that helps build a bridge between small-scale sustainable producers and their customers.

were around long before the local food movement rose to popularity. They enable farmers to work together as a community, and they help small-scale producers to better compete with the supermarket distribution available to large-scale producers.

Grass farm. A farm that focuses on pasture-raised food.

Pasture. A grassy open area managed for grazing livestock and poultry. Well-managed pasture builds rich topsoil.

Permaculture. An agricultural system that models itself after nature to create a self-sustaining ecosystem that produces food. Australians Bill Mollison and David Holmgren coined the term "permaculture" in 1978, but similar techniques have been used by horticulturalists and small-scale farmers across the globe. Permaculture typically mixes livestock and poultry with pasture and trees, and uses little or no tillage.

Topsoil. The upper layer of the ground that, when healthy, is teeming with life, rich in minerals, and a fertile home for plant life. All agriculture depends on vibrant topsoil.

How Does 'Local Food' Incorporate These Ideas?

After poring through all these terms, you might be wondering, if the whole issue is as convoluted as this lexicon implies, why go with a simple word like "local" to describe it? The national impulse toward a better food system is not just about health, nutrition, environmental responsibility, job security, economic equality, or animal welfare, but *all of these together*. Does the word "local," by itself, really capture the complexity of this issue?

If you're looking for a single attribute that embodies all these positive ideas, local is probably the best choice. In many cases, just by virtue of being local, the food you buy will meet many of the other criteria I've mentioned. Whether it's strictly organic or not, food obtained from a local small producer is more likely to be grown using sustainable, low-impact methods—and because they're in your area, you can visit the farm and see for yourself whether or not those methods meet your requirements. If you get your food directly from the farmer or, at least, from the local organization that got it from the

I've Heard of the Local Food Movement, But What's the 'Slow Food' Movement?

Italian activist Carlo Petrini coined the term "slow food" in 1986 to refer to the antithesis of "fast food." Petrini advocates a diet of foods that are grown locally, prepared within the context of a regional cuisine, and savored at leisure.

farmer, it won't have had the opportunity to undergo a lot of processing. And whenever you buy from growers in your area, you're supporting your local economy.

Organic farmer Nick Maravell explains that buying local food is the only way to put the farmer in direct contact with the customer. "To the extent you do that," he says, "both the farmer and the customer benefit." In his more than three decades of farming, he has seen that customers who visit farms develop an appreciation of the land and are more likely to take action to preserve natural resources. He also claims that supporting local and regional farms is the best way for consumers to assure they're getting safe, healthy, fresh food. "Grocery store cashiers don't know much about the products they're selling. Ask a farmer, and you get the *real* answer. The relationship between consumer and farmer is the only thing that can't be co-opted by larger corporate concerns," he says.

Pumpkin Loaf

2 cups all-purpose flour

1 cup cooked mashed pumpkin

1 cup honey or light brown sugar

1/2 cup cream

2 eggs

1/4 cup butter

1 teaspoon vanilla extract

1 teaspoon baking powder

1/2 teaspoon baking soda

1 teaspoon cinnamon

1/4 teaspoon nutmeg

Soften the butter and beat in the pumpkin, vanilla extract, cream, and honey or sugar. Whip the eggs separately and then mix them into the butter mixture. In a separate bowl, combine the flour, baking soda, baking powder, cinnamon, and nutmeg. Slowly add the dry mixture to the butter mixture while stirring. Pour the batter into a greased loaf pan. Bake at 325 degrees for 45 minutes, or until the middle is no longer jiggly.

6

Local vs. Industrial

A Side-by-Side Comparison

It's not what you look at that matters, it's what you see. —*Henry David Thoreau*

That organic stuff, is it really worth the price?"

This is the inevitable question that comes up when I talk to students about alternatives to industrial food. The person asking expects a simple answer: yes, organics are worth paying extra; no, organics are money wasted. I pause, and take a deep breath, knowing that the answer I'm about to give them will be far longer and more complicated than they want.

Something in our culture leads us to think in this monochromatic way, particularly about what we eat. We've ridden the wave of so many food fads, each one meant to do one single, spectacular thing for our health. Oat bran will fix our hearts, antioxidants will halt aging, and omega-3 fatty acids will transform us into geniuses.

I wish it were that simple.

By now, you've probably noticed that the common thread running throughout this book is the idea that food is complex. The methods by which it's produced, prepared, marketed, and sold have impacts on many aspects of our lives. We can't get a complete picture if we're focusing only on nutrition, or environmental impact, or economic concerns. To really understand food, we need to take a holistic approach.

My answer to the students' question is that buying organic food is *one* step toward better health and sustainable production. It removes potentially harmful chemicals from the environment and the human food chain, and yes, in a few studies, it has been found to be more nutritious. But deciding whether or not to buy organic is only part of the issue. We also need to be

Holism

The recognition that any part of a system cannot be properly understood without reference to the whole.

thinking about many other factors in order to make an informed decision about our food.

In this chapter, I'll compare twenty-one industrially produced foods to their local, organic, or small-scale-production alternatives, and in some cases where a homemade or homegrown option exists, I'll offer that as a substitute. I obtained the information in this chapter by reading labels, visiting company websites, and in most cases, buying, preparing, tasting, and experimenting with these foods. I'll compare these items by cost, convenience, nutrition, and environmental impact. I've included the actual prices of certain items as noted at the time of this writing, so naturally, any prices you see listed here are subject to change.

Before we get into it, I need to throw in one small caveat: comparing one nonindustrial item with its industrial counterpart is a little misleading, because doing this implies that you'd simply be selecting the nonindustrial equivalent of the exact same thing. In most cases, breaking your dependency on the industrial system means choosing completely different foods. You're swapping patented, highly processed, overly packaged products containing several dozen ingredients, only a fraction of which really qualify as food, for items that have a half dozen ingredients or less, little or no packaging, and many of which need no label.

Let's start with the stuff that fits the purest definition of food: single-ingredient items, grown on farms, sold in something approximating their natural state. We'll compare organic with nonorganic, heirloom variety with supermarket variety, seasonal with out-of-season, small-scale with large-scale production, and grass fed (pastured) with confinement fed (CAFO).

Farm Goods: Organic vs. Nonorganic

In Chapter 5, we defined organic agriculture as a method that grows food without synthetic chemical inputs. It ensures that the plant or animal was grown without artificial herbicides, pesticides, fertilizers, hormones, or other pharmaceuticals. Just because an item's label bears the logo "USDA Organic" does not automatically make it local, humanely, or sustainably produced, grown on a small scale, more nutritious, or better tasting. Advocates of wiser food production might say that organic is necessary, but not sufficient. It's an important part of the holistic equation, but only part.

Organic vs. Nonorganic: Milk

In spite of American culture's long love affair with dairy products, and the USDA's Choose My Plate recommendation that a serving of dairy be included in every meal, scientific evidence has been quietly accumulating that call the benefits of milk into question and point to health risks associated with it.

We've long been told that milk is essential to our diets, particularly because of its calcium. Yet, according to the Harvard School of Public Health, the daily calcium we need can also be obtained from a diet rich in fresh vegetables, especially dark leafy greens.

According to the Physicians Committee for Responsible Medicine, high dairy consumption has been linked to obesity as well as the onset of certain cancers, particularly breast and prostate cancer. Most milk products are high in fat, and even skim milk contains cholesterol. The Physicians Committee for Responsible Medicine also cites studies in which traces of chemical residues, such as dioxin and polychlorinated biphenyls, have been found in milk. Recently, consumers have become concerned over the effects on human health of the recombinant bovine growth hormone (rBGH), routinely fed to CAFO dairy cows to speed up milk production.

Will drinking *organic* milk help you avoid these risks? Some of them. Cows in organic USDA Certified Organic dairies are not given rBGH, and their feed has not been sprayed with synthetic pesticides or herbicides. Unfortunately, organic milk has as much fat and cholesterol as nonorganic milk.

When you leave the CAFO entirely and seek out milk that is not only organic, but also from cows fed on their natural diet of grass, you get an additional benefit: grass-fed cows have five times as much conjugated linoleic acid in their milk than that of industrial feed-lot dairy cows. This unsaturated fat appears to offer protective benefits to the heart and may actually aid in weight loss.

The USDA now also requires that organic dairies give their cows access to pasture for at least 120 days each year. Dairies that specialize in milk from grass-fed cattle often give their cows far more grass time than this. The nutritional data seems to suggest that the more access to pasture a dairy cow is granted, the more nutritious her milk.

Convenience. Today, in most urban and suburban areas, you can find organic brands of milk in the dairy case alongside nonorganics, making them just as convenient to obtain. More convenient still, many small local organic dairies offer home delivery. To find one in your area, visit LocalHarvest at www.localharvest.org, type in your zip code, and search "organic milk." If you're looking for *grass-fed* or *pastured* organic milk, those words will appear in the product description. If you don't see them, you can usually assume that the milk is from the industrial system.

Taste. In an online article dated January 18, 2012, the *Huffington Post* published the results of a taste test performed by twenty-three of its editors, who tasted samples of both organic and nonorganic milk. According to the article, 53 percent could identify which was organic and which was not; 56 percent preferred the taste of organic milk. In my own experience, in the taste department, what really makes milk taste the way it did when I was a kid has less to do with whether it's organic and everything to do with how much time the cows spend on pasture. Milk from grass-fed cows tastes better.

Nutrition. In December 2013, in the online journal *PLoS ONE*, a research team from Washington State University released the findings of their study comparing the omega-3 fatty acids in organic milk with those in regular milk. After comparing more than 400 samples over an eighteen-month period, they found that organic milk had a 2.3 ratio of harmful omega-6 fatty acids to beneficial omega-3s, where regular milk's ratio came in at 5.8. In other words, organic milk had less of the bad stuff and more of the good stuff.

Economic impact. A survey of grocery store chains in my area revealed that organic milk from large producers cost an average of $1.86 more per half-gallon than nonorganic. Why the price difference? Organic farmers must adhere to a different, and often more costly, set of standards.

Also, CAFO cows get that turbocharged boost to their milk production in the form of recombinant bovine growth hormone. Hormone-free organic dairy cows produce at the speed nature allows. The more productive the cows, the lower the price of their milk. But the real question here is *at what ultimate cost do we enjoy super-low-priced milk?*

Environmental impact. Just because milk is labeled organic doesn't mean all organic milk has the same environmental footprint. Many organic brands found in national supermarket chains don't give their cows recombinant bovine growth hormone and the animals' feed is pesticide free, but the cows are still raised in large-scale operations and their milk is shipped long distances to markets in multiple states.

Substitution. My own preference has been to virtually eliminate milk from my diet, though I do eat cheese and butter. In place of milk, I drink unsweetened organic soy milk, which avoids all the health risks associated with milk that I mentioned previously, has zero grams of cholesterol, and provides me with the same 30 percent of my daily calcium as milk and seven grams of protein, compared with the eight I'd get in milk. (To be entirely fair, I have to note that the USDA's Choose My Plate program does include soy milk under its list of dairy options, but it's one choice among the twenty-three others that are based on cow's milk.) A number of studies have been published in recent decades that suggest soy protein in extremely large quantities—as in, quarts per day—can have detrimental health effects, but trust me, I don't drink *that* much. Also, most of the nonorganic soy in the U.S. has been genetically modified to be resistant to the herbicide glyphosate (aka Roundup).

How does soy milk compare with cow's milk, price wise? A half-gallon of regular milk costs about $2.39, the same amount of organic milk costs $4.29, and the equivalent amount of organic soy milk costs $2.99. For sixty cents more, I enjoy all the health benefits and avoid the risks.

Oh, and one more aside before we leave the discussion about soy milk: over the past six months, I've been buying three half-gallons of organic soy milk per week, alongside the four half-gallons of cow's milk my husband orders from our local dairy. Every week, my sons and husband use up all the soy milk long before the cow's milk is gone. Why? They say it's because the soy milk tastes better.

How Do You Milk a Soybean?

Have you ever wondered what it takes to get a milk-like substance from soybeans? Turns out, it's easy. Soak dry soybeans in water overnight, grind them with water (you can do this in a blender, food processor, or in some juicers), and pour the liquid through a cheese-cloth or strainer.

Organic vs. Nonorganic: Lettuce

If you decide not to go full-out organic, but instead choose to buy some of your produce organic and some of it not, lettuce is a good item to add to the organic list. Any leafy vegetable, including spinach, kale, cabbage, and bok choi, might well make the "buy organic" list, because if we buy them in nonorganic form, we're probably eating leaves that have come in direct contact with sprayed pesticides and herbicides. Growers thoroughly wash their leaves of pesticide residues before passing them along to consumers, but many shoppers would prefer that these chemicals never come in direct contact with things they plan to put in their bodies.

Convenience. Many CSAs and farm delivery services offer organic lettuce on a weekly basis year-round. Farmers can grow lettuce in hoop-houses throughout the year in all but the coldest zones of the U.S., though the nutritional density and flavor appear to diminish a bit when greens are grown in winter.

Taste. Organic lettuce from the supermarket tastes no different to me than nonorganic. The real taste difference is between the store-bought lettuce and the tender baby lettuce I can grow in my yard during cool weather or in an indoor window box in winter. My own crisp, sweet, homegrown leaves taste of minerals and cool spring rain.

Nutrition. Is organic lettuce more nutritious than nonorganic lettuce? As I discussed in Chapter 3, it's really the soil health, not the organic method, that makes the greatest nutritional difference. We've yet to see enough independent research *asking the right questions* to really settle this debate. Has anyone compared industrially grown vegetables with those grown in a carefully managed permaculture environment, where soil health is the number one priority?

Another factor that influences the nutritional value of lettuce, as well as any other vegetable, is its freshness. The longer any produce sits around, the more its nutritional components degrade. As a general rule, the farther the distance between where it's grown and where it's eaten, the longer it's spent sitting in a shipping container. So maybe we shouldn't be asking "organic vs. nonorganic?" so much as "shipped vs. local?" And of course, if it's true that the fresher the produce, the denser the nutrition, then the freshest lettuce of all is the kind you snipped from your window box this morning.

Economic impact. At the supermarket, a head of regular romaine lettuce costs $1.99, but on the day I surveyed prices, organic romaine lettuce cost only fifty cents more. The local delivery service from which we get most of our produce will deliver a head of organic romaine lettuce for about $3.25. For $1.26 more than at the supermarket, we get leaves that have never been adulterated with chemicals, *plus* the convenience of not having to drive to the store for them.

Before we leave the subject of lettuce, I'd like to add a word about packaged salad kits. Here's where the convenience of processing costs you big time: a head of lettuce weighs one to two pounds on average, so when you buy your lettuce by the pound, this translates to $1.00 to $1.50 per pound. A bagged salad kit will run you $2.99 to $4.99, even though you're getting only seven to twelve ounces of lettuce per bag. That runs the average cost per head up to $6.00 or $6.50 per pound, and most of those salad kits are not even organic. All you need to do is choose the whole organic head of romaine instead, invest the thirty seconds it takes to *chop your own lettuce*, and you've just *saved* about $3.00 by buying organic!

Organic vs. Nonorganic: Bananas

If you purchase bananas anywhere in the United States, odds are you're buying imports. It's possible to grow bananas in Florida and Hawaii, but the majority of bananas grown on U.S. soil are for small niche markets.

Assuming you're still going to buy bananas, even though they're probably imported, would you go for the organic ones? Many guides to organic foods recommend that, if you can only buy some of your produce organic, you could skip organic bananas because the inedible peel protects the fruit inside from direct contact with herbicides and pesticides.

Convenience, taste, and nutrition. At a large supermarket in a suburban area, getting your hands on an organic banana may be as easy as buying the regular kind. As far as flavor, I have yet to meet the person who can distinguish an organic banana from a nonorganic one by taste alone. Likewise with nutrition: the nutritional profiles for organic and nonorganic bananas appear to be about the same.

Economic impact. In terms of your family's economy, an organic banana will run you about ten cents more. But in the broader picture of the global economy, an important trend is afoot. Many banana farmers in developing countries have found advocates in the Fair Trade movement, which promotes equitable trading conditions and living wages for farmers, and attempts to put an end to corporate exploitation. You'll know you've found a banana from a grower who participates in this program if it bears the Certified Fair Trade sticker.

Environmental impact. As with any comparison between organic and nonorganic farming methods, the main difference is in the fact that organic growers don't use synthetic herbicides, pesticides, or other chemical inputs. Historically, large-scale banana farming has had a negative environmental impact because of monoculturing and other industrial practices. Even an organic banana farm extracts a hefty toll from its environment if it grows its fruit through large-scale monoculture.

The other major environmental strike against bananas is that most are shipped to us from other countries, so their environmental footprint is large because of the miles they've logged in getting to you. If you live in a semi-tropical part of our country or have a heated greenhouse, you can grow your own. Otherwise, the bananas your family consumes are likely to be pretty well traveled.

Farm Goods: In Season vs. Out of Season

Our generation is accustomed to getting almost any kind of fruit or vegetable we want at any time of year. Most of us are unaware that this year-round availability is historically abnormal. A hundred years ago, almost everyone ate foods in season by necessity. Today, many people are eating seasonally because produce in season is cheaper, tastier, and because it's local, leaves a daintier environmental footprint.

It's entirely possible to feed your family well on local produce all winter long in any part of the United States, even Alaska. It's just not something you can do without a little forethought. From May to September, in most of the country, all the locavores are living large. But the local eater knows that when October approaches, she'd better buy up the last of the winter squashes at the Saturday farmers' market, freeze and can a few things, and throw an extra layer of mulch on the fall spinach crop in the backyard, because local pickings are about to get slim.

In Season vs. Out of Season: Asparagus, Zucchini, Apples

Over the past few decades, we've grown accustomed to eating these three items year-round. We expect them to be available anytime we wander into a supermarket. A generation ago, all three of these foods would have been considered seasonal specialties. Supermarket shoppers today are hardly aware that produce has a season. For the most part, we simply don't think about where our food comes from and what it takes to grow it. We may know, on some antiseptic, intellectual level that zucchinis don't grow in cold weather, but as we eagerly buy a half-dozen of them for a New Year's Eve lasagna, it simply doesn't compute.

Convenience. Many people argue that importing fruits and vegetables means more flavor and variety year-round. But produce that has come from thousands of miles away has often spent a great deal of time sitting around in shipping containers, all the while losing flavor, texture, and nutrients. Those of us who are used to obtaining our produce from supermarkets think bland and mushy is the way fruits and vegetables are supposed to be. Who wants to eat that stuff, when the fast food joint across the road sells a cheeseburger for the same price as an apple?

Taste. The simple reality is that humans tend to eat what tastes good, and produce that has been sitting for weeks or months in a crate *doesn't*. I'd submit to you that the average American eats far fewer fruits and vegetables today than she did a hundred years ago, because so much of today's supermarket produce tastes like candle wax, while processed food is expressly designed to produce an outrageous flavor burst on the tongue.

But fresh, local fruits and vegetables *in season* are so vibrantly flavorful that even the laboratory-concocted jolts of artificial flavor in processed foods can't compete. If you truly want to understand the difference seasonality makes to the taste of fruits and vegetables, there's only one way to find out, and you can't get it from a book. Asparagus is at its peak in April or May for most of the United States, though it can be ready as early as February in southern climates and as late as June in northern ones. Zucchini, a warm-weather-loving fruit, is at its peak from June through August in most of the U.S. In very warm climates such as Florida, zucchini does best in spring and fall, as it dislikes extreme heat. The peak season for most varieties of apples, regardless of agricultural zone, is September through November. A few early varieties are ready to harvest in July. Even though apples can store well for up to a year, they're a totally different experience when eaten fresh-picked.

Nutrition. When the question of nutrition arises, people usually compare organic with nonorganic, small production with large, frozen with fresh, or one variety with another. But what really makes the difference, in both taste and nutrition, is how long it's been since the food was harvested. The fresher the food, the higher the nutritional content. This is the real secret behind the goodness of seasonal produce: it was *alive and growing* just hours or days before you eat it.

Fruit and vegetable specialist Dr. Diane M. Barrett, of the University of California, Davis, recently reviewed the literature comparing the nutritional properties of fresh, frozen, and canned products. She found that the nutritional profiles of fresh fruits and vegetables can degrade significantly within a week after harvest. After seven days in cool storage, green peas lose 15 percent of their nutrients, and green beans lose 77 percent.

Dr. Barrett explains that vitamins A and C, the B vitamins, and nutrients such as lycopene are sensitive to heat and light. Many nutrients are affected by exposure to oxygen, water, and acidity levels. Mechanical harvesting may also cause nutrients to degrade because it causes more damage to the tissues of fruits and vegetables than handpicking.

If I tried to push the data in this survey to the max, I'd probably conclude that the most nutritious way to eat produce is to pick it by hand at the peak of season and eat it raw on the spot. Because this isn't the most practical way to obtain three square meals year-round, the best bet for maximizing nutrition is to habitually eat fresh local in-season produce *as often as possible*.

Economic impact. At the supermarket in early winter, one Fuji apple costs 99 cents. Locally grown Fuji apples from a farm in Smithsburg, Md., cost $3.25 for three, about eight cents more per apple. But not included in this price is the fact that the apples arrived on my doorstep courtesy of our local delivery service, which saved me the cost of gas, as well as the intangible expense of my time and energy, because I didn't have to drive to the grocery store.

Environmental impact. Anytime a crate of fruit or vegetables is transported anywhere by something that runs on fossil fuel, it produces a negative effect on the environment. The farther it is shipped, the greater the impact. Commercial produce moves to market using one or more of these means: truck, train, boat, or aircraft, and every one of these forms of transport runs on fossil fuels. They also require roads, rail beds, bridges, ports, landing strips, and other infrastructure, all of which leave an environmental footprint. The asparagus, zucchini, and apples you pick from your backyard garden make the tiniest impact, and if you grow them by methods that enhance the local ecosystem, the overall impact is a positive one. The same produce from a grower within fifty miles of you makes a slightly larger footprint, but even the size of that print can be reduced by having *one* delivery truck make the neighborhood rounds, instead of hundreds of individual shoppers driving their vehicles to grocery stores.

Farm Goods: Heirloom Variety vs. Supermarket Variety

In a supermarket, the greatest variety is found in the processed food aisles. There's comparatively little to be had in the produce section. A whole generation of Americans—the ones who, when you ask them where food comes from, reply, "the grocery store"—don't realize that produce comes in more varieties than three kinds of tomatoes, four types of lettuce, and two sorts of potato. A century ago, farmers and gardeners routinely grew *hundreds* of different varieties of produce.

Few American grocery store shoppers are aware that the varieties of fruits and vegetables to which they're accustomed were developed specifically for a mass market. Supermarket produce developers wanted a tomato that ripened evenly and could sit on a shelf for a long time. The gene they cultivated that causes even-ripening also causes the fruit to taste like a soggy paper towel. I'm certain that food scientists are working on this, so it may not always be the case. But so far, not even the most talented wizard-chemist

Growing Harvests, Shrinking Variety

The domestication of plants and animals has allowed for a dramatic increase in human populations worldwide. Anywhere there's arable land, farmers can feed a far larger population than even the most skilled hunters and gatherers could. But a growing reliance on food production has spelled a shrinking variety of species available for use as food, because farmers end up favoring crops and animals with the highest yields and ignoring all the other choices. The result is an ever-narrowing range of resources.

In the past, human beings have found sustenance in more than ten thousand species of plant foods. Today, we cultivate hardly more than 150 species, and of those, farmers worldwide rely on just twelve species for 80 percent of the world's crops.

Why is this problematic? Because an overreliance on a small number of species makes a population vulnerable to famine. It has happened within the recent past. During the mid 1800s, Ireland suffered a collapse of its potato crop because of a catastrophic blight. According to some estimates, the death toll from this famine may have run as high as one million.

can make a supermarket tomato taste like the ones fresh-picked from my granddaddy's garden.

Before the rise of modern grocery stores, when people still bought most of their food whole and unprocessed from small markets or farmers, and when most people grew at least a little bit of their own food, more people knew that vegetables and fruits came in dozens, even hundreds, of varieties.

Our supermarket-dependent society is driving hundreds of these fine old heirloom varieties to the brink of extinction. This is too bad for a number of reasons. First, many heirlooms were cultivated to take advantage of specific growing conditions. Second, most of these old varieties were bred not for conformity or shipability but for flavor. Third, a geneticist will tell you that the key to the survival of any species is genetic diversity, which is precisely what we're losing by forfeiting hundreds of heirloom varieties in favor of a handful of supermarket varieties. Fourth—and we're now just discovering this—some of those old-time varieties have far more nutritional density than their supermarket counterparts.

I picked the tomato for this particular comparison because no other vegetable has its Jekyll-and-Hyde reputation for supermarket drabness and backyard garden charisma. The tomato is the vegetable ambassador for the local food movement.

Heirloom Variety vs. Supermarket Variety: Tomatoes

Big-chain grocery stores seldom carry heirloom varieties of anything. Many farmers' market vendors specialize in heirlooms, but in most parts of the U.S., they're not an option year-round, because they have specific growing seasons.

The best way to experience the endless quirky variety of heirloom tomatoes is to grow them. Baker Creek Heirloom Seed Company's 2014 catalog boasts more than 1,500 types of rare, non-GMO seeds, including 190 varieties of tomato, which they categorize as green, orange, pink, purple, black, brown, red, white, and bi-color. A packet of any one of these will only set you back about $2.50.

Convenience. Let's be completely honest. Gardening will never be as convenient as going to the supermarket. But you could reframe it as a trade-off. This year, you might decide to ditch the fantasy football league, unplug the game console, or log off of social media, and instead take up a hobby that yields delicious, nutritious food for your family. Just a suggestion.

Taste. I've never met a supermarket tomato that I got along with, organic or not. I simply don't buy them, even during tomato season. I'd rather forgo fresh tomatoes entirely when they're not in season. It makes me appreciate them that much more when their season comes around. The taste of an heirloom tomato, fresh-picked from my own garden in the middle of summer, sliced and sprinkled with a little salt and pepper: that alone is a reason to go on living.

Nutrition. Because supermarket products are bred primarily for fast growth, shipability, and long shelf life, and heirloom varieties are bred primarily for regional compatibility and fresh eating, it seems like a no brainer that heirlooms would contain more nutrients. But as yet, there have been few rigorous independent studies comparing the nutritional profiles of supermarket-bred produce to that of heirloom varieties. So, to answer the question of nutrition, I put together information from two sources: the USDA's nutritional analysis of a supermarket tomato and an heirloom seed company's own independent research.

Baker Creek Heirloom Seed Company funded a study comparing the nutritional profiles of several of its tomato varieties, which they published in their 2014 seed catalog. Its nutritional superstars included the Black Krim, with 606 international units of vitamin A, and the Indigo Apple, with 39.55 milligrams of vitamin C. By comparison, according to the USDA, the plum Roma tomato, a common grocery store offering, contains 516 international units of A and 8.5 milligrams of C.

If the supermarket plum Roma were placed on Baker Creek's nutritional scale, it might fall somewhere in the middle or bottom third of the nutritional continuum. But, keeping in mind that the most nutritious produce is whatever's freshest, the only remaining question is which one is more likely to be eaten fresher: the supermarket Roma that may have been out of the field as long as a month, or the heirloom tomato you picked from your garden this morning?

Economic impact. Off-season, a nonorganic beefsteak tomato from the supermarket costs about $1.49. The organic equivalent costs up to $2.29. Interestingly enough, when I priced a supermarket's offering of grape tomatoes, I found that an organic pint and a nonorganic pint cost the same: $3.99. In season, fresh heirloom tomatoes from local farmers cost *about the same* as the ones from the supermarket, and the ones you grow in your garden, the absolute best tomatoes in the world, cost pennies per pound.

Heirloom Fruits and Veggies Are Bred for Taste

I asked Kathy McFarland of Baker Creek Heirloom Seeds why their customers prefer to plant heirlooms. She said, "Heirloom varieties taste better than hybrid and genetically modified varieties because they have been selected, bred, and grown for many generations based on the tastes of home gardeners and independent farmers." Kathy and the rest of the Baker Creek staff feel that it's important to keep heirloom varieties from going extinct. "The diversity of heirlooms adds interest, nutrition, and variety to our diet."

Aside from their flavor, the other thing that's easy to love about heirlooms is their colorful variety of names. Baker Creek's 2014 catalog features varieties such as Greasy Grits beans, Dragon's Egg cucumbers, Little Sailor eggplants, Indian Cream Cobra melons, Candy Roaster squash, and Tommy Toe tomatoes.

Farm Goods: Small-Scale Production vs. Large-Scale Production

Although an economist might be quick to extol the virtues of scale in any commercial venture, bigger isn't always better. In large-scale farming operations, everything is designed for high volume and speed, from the variety of plant or animal grown to the means by which they're processed. The industrial system produces an enormous amount of food that can be sold to the consumer at relatively low cost. But large-scale farming, which the USDA Economic Research Service defines as an agricultural operation that makes more than $250,000 in annual sales, nearly always relies on techniques such as monoculture and confined animal feeding operations. This system seems efficient in the short run, but in fact, it's feeding today's eaters at the expense of tomorrow's.

Small-scale producers are more likely to practice farming techniques that mimic natural cycles. Small farms require fewer inputs from off-farm sources in the form of animal feeds, fertilizers, pharmaceuticals, and other chemicals. A farmer who composts his livestock's manure doesn't need to buy synthetic fertilizers. If he also grows most of his animals' feed on-site, he doesn't have to ship in hay or grain. If his animals live in conditions that allow for the expression of their natural behaviors, they're less likely to get ill, so there's no need to feed them routine antibiotics. Bugs and larvae are controlled, at least in part, by hungry poultry, so there's less need for pesticides. When crops and animals are frequently rotated to fresh sites, they stay one step ahead of many pests. Not all small-scale farmers follow nature-inspired practices such as these, but you'd be hard-pressed to find a large operation that does.

Small-Scale Production vs. Large-Scale Production: Pork

Pigs have gotten a bad rap as filthy animals, and nothing I say in my classroom has been able to change that. When we talk about the deeper cultural rationale behind kosher laws and the Muslim prohibition against eating pork, the common misconception is that these laws exist to prevent people from eating a dirty animal. But the perception we Americans have of pigs wallowing in their own excrement comes from confinement practices we've come to think of as normal. Free-range pigs are comparatively clean.

So, if pigs aren't inherently dirty, what's behind these dietary laws?

According to anthropologist Marvin Harris, the cultural prohibition against eating pigs first arose in historically arid regions, where agriculture is difficult. It has more to do with the fact that, as omnivores, these animals compete with humans for the same food sources, so that in the most marginal environments, they're not practical. Yet, no matter how hard I hit the note about the cleanliness of pigs, when this question appears on an exam, most students still answer that the prohibition against pigs exists because they're dirty.

In less arid regions, pigs are welcome complements to a diversified farm. Historically, people have turned their pigs loose to forage for themselves on wooded lands, to be hunted and butchered in the autumn. Their rooting aerates soil and gives dormant seeds a chance to sprout. Their trampling can keep vegetation growth at bay. In Spain, the ham that fetches the highest prices comes from black Iberico pigs that have fed themselves on acorns. The meat of acorn-fed pigs is described as exceptionally lean and intensely flavorful.

Pork from large-scale industrial hog farms is quite different. Never in their lives do these animals root around in cool forests. They spend the whole of their existence in enclosures too small to allow them much movement. According to animal behavior expert Temple Grandin, the frustration and understimulation these highly intelligent animals experience during their confinement causes them to chew one another's tails. They are fed a corn-based diet to fatten them quickly for slaughter. Unless it's labeled otherwise, this is the default meat you're getting whenever you buy pork from a grocery store.

Convenience. Free-range pork is difficult to find. Although CAFO-raised pork is ubiquitous in every supermarket, you'll probably have to approach a pork farmer, CSA, or distributor to obtain free-range pork.

Nutrition. I have yet to locate an independent study that fairly and accurately compares the nutritional profiles of CAFO and free-range pork. Many farmers strongly assert that pastured animals produce leaner meat as a result of moving around more, and that a forage-based diet builds more nutritional density in the meat.

Economic impact. I have yet to find pork from small producers for anything close to the same price as CAFO pork. A December 2013 price survey found supermarket pork shoulder at $2.49 per pound, while the same item from a local small farm cost $5.49 per pound. How do you handle a price difference like this? You could relegate pork to the status of occasional luxury, to be savored in small quantities at special meals, which is what a nutritionist would probably advise you to do, anyway.

Environmental impact. Hog CAFOs are notoriously harsh on their environments. Laura B. Delind's 1998 study of a 5,000-hog farming operation in Parma, Michigan, published in Thu and Durrenberger's *Pigs, Profits, and Rural Communities*, revealed that after the facility opened in 1983, fish disappeared from local creeks, airborne particles contaminated swimming pools, and the stench drove businesses out of town and caused real estate prices to drop.

By contrast, free-range hogs, responsibly managed, may actually benefit the ecology of a small farm because their trampling and rooting controls weeds and aerates soil. They're also an efficient means to handle kitchen scraps because they'll eat anything we eat. Their manure doesn't have to be dumped into lagoons. It can be composted to fertilize crops. The same stuff that's a health hazard in one scenario becomes a boon in the other.

Farm Goods: Pastured vs. CAFO

A hundred years ago, it was normal for meat, milk, and eggs to come from pastured animals. Today, the vast majority of the pork, beef, chicken, turkey, eggs, and dairy that Americans consume are the products of CAFOs, concentrated animal feeding operations. Meat, milk, and eggs from animals raised on pasture, once the norm, are now considered boutique foods for niche markets. Because informed eaters seek them out, pastured animal products are almost guaranteed to be labeled as such. No meat, dairy, or egg producer ever puts the word "CAFO" on its packaging!

Pastured vs. CAFO: Eggs
Many CAFO opponents argue that the cruelest treatment of any confined animals is that given to laying hens. These birds spend a lifetime in cages too small to allow them to spread a wing. They never see the inside of a nesting

box and instead are forced to lay their eggs into collection troughs. Their lives are painful and brief.

"Cage free" farming doesn't entirely solve the problem. Uncaged laying hens may still be raised indoors on corn-based feed and may still never have the luxury of exercising many of their natural behaviors.

In contrast, truly pasture-raised eggs come from hens that roam at will from mobile henhouses, which are regularly moved to fresh grass. They browse through foliage for bugs and other tasty morsels. These animals can express their natural behaviors and suffer far less stress than their indoor sisters. If this is how you prefer your eggs, you'll need to look for the words "grass fed" or "pastured" on the carton.

Convenience. Although your large-chain supermarket will probably offer many options such as "cage free" and "cruelty free," they probably won't offer truly pasture-raised eggs. For these, you will need to visit a co-op or farmers' market or arrange to purchase them from a local grass farmer.

Taste. Pastured eggs taste far more vibrant and "eggy" than CAFO eggs. Their firm yolks exhibit a bright golden-orange hue.

Nutrition. Lately, as I've surveyed the eggs on offer at grocery stores, I've wondered, why the obsession with eggs from "vegetarian-fed hens"? Chickens are not normally vegetarians. They're omnivores like us. Chickens raised without sufficient protein in their diets develop all kinds of disabling disorders. I suspect what's fueling this trend is fear that agricultural waste proteins may be added to the hens' feed, and this kind of feed may be contaminated or may produce higher cholesterol eggs. But vegetarian hens never eat the one ingredient that gives their eggs the greatest nutritional boost: *bugs!*

Hens that forage aggressively for tasty wigglies produce nutritionally superior eggs. A 2007 study by *Mother Earth News* comparing CAFO with free-range eggs found that pasture-raised eggs could contain as much as two-thirds more vitamin A, three times more vitamin E, two times more omega-3 fatty acids, and seven times more beta carotene, while carrying one-third less cholesterol and one-fourth less saturated fat.

Economic impact. A dozen grade A large eggs from the supermarket cost, on average, $1.89 to $2.39. Any specialty eggs, such as "certified humane,"

USDA Nutritional Analysis

NUTRIENT	GRASS-FED BEEF	COMMODITY BEEF
Protein	19.42 g	17.37 g
Fat	12.73 g	17.07 g
Calcium	12 mg	7 mg
Iron	1.99 mg	1.69 mg
Magnesium	19 mg	17 mg
Phosphorus	175 mg	122 mg
Potassium	289 mg	246 mg
Sodium	68 mg	57 mg
Zinc	4.55 mg	3.59 mg
Thiamin	0.049 mg	0.056 mg
Riboflavin	0.154 mg	0.232 mg
Niacin	4.818 mg	4.207 mg
Vitamin B6	0.355 mg	0.241 mg
Folate	6 mcg	7 mcg
Vitamin B12	1.97 mcg	1.91 mcg
Cholesterol	62 mg	69 mg

According to the USDA's nutritional analysis, grass-fed ground beef is higher in protein, calcium, and several other key nutrients, and lower in cholesterol and total fat, than commodity ground beef.

"cage free," "free range," or "organic" may tack on an additional two to four dollars. Truly pastured eggs from small producers vary in price. At last check, the most expensive pastured eggs I could find sold for $6.38 a dozen, the cheapest for $3.50.

Pastured vs. CAFO: Beef

If you've seen Robert Kenner's film *Food, Inc.* or read Eric Schlosser's *Fast Food Nation*, you may be eager to switch to pastured beef because it's less likely to be exposed to the unsanitary conditions and hasty processing you saw portrayed in the movie and book. If you've got a good understanding of the role that healthy soil plays in producing nutritionally dense and flavorful foods, you might seek out grass-fed beef for these reasons as well.

Convenience. Upscale supermarkets now carry selections of grass-fed beef, but they're much more expensive than the ordinary kind, because in that venue, "grass fed" seems to come under the umbrella of "boutique foods." If you don't mind the inconvenience of a drive out to your local grass farm, and especially if you're prepared to buy in bulk and store multiple beef cuts in your freezer, a farmer will probably give you a better price on pasture-raised beef than your grocery store will.

Taste. To my taste buds, grass-fed ground beef is far more flavorful than the CAFO equivalent, but not everyone finds the difference to their liking. A friend who switched to grass-fed beef on my recommendation reported that her family complained about the taste. However, we once fed grilled grass-fed beef burgers to our sons' teenage friends during a backyard barbecue to rave reviews.

Nutrition. I compared the Nutritional Facts labels on CAFO and grass-fed beef and found that CAFO beef has more calories, fat, trans fat, and cholesterol. Grass-fed beef has more protein and calcium. The USDA's online nutritional database, ndb.nal.usda.gov, lists the nutritional profiles for grass-fed and commodity beef. Grass-fed beef had higher amounts of nine beneficial nutrients than its commodity counterpart.

Economic impact. In mid December 2013, the cheapest supermarket ground beef, which, of course, came from a CAFO, was $2.87 per pound. A pound of grass-fed ground beef raised in Florida cost $7.99 from our local supermarket. At that same time, our local dairy would deliver a pound of locally raised, grass-fed, no-hormone ground beef to our door for $4.89.

Environmental impact. Many environmentalists have spoken out strongly against beef production. They argue that it takes numerous pounds of feed and hundreds of gallons of water to produce one pound of beef. They claim that beef production ties up arable land that might otherwise be tilled for crops. Anti-beef advocates argue that we could grow the same number of calories from plant sources with far fewer inputs.

At first it seems hard to fault their logic—until you consider that not all land is equally suited for tillage. Pastured beef makes the most sense in regions where growing row crops is less viable. It also makes sense, from the perspective of diversified farming, to raise a small number of cattle on parts of a farm that aren't as good for crops: hilly areas, for instance. To many environmentalists who value soil health, pasturing animals makes more sense than plowing and tilling for row crops, because they cause less disturbance to the soil.

If we relegated cattle to those ecosystems and microclimates where they made sense, and raised them on the proper scale for the given environment, beef production would make a much lighter impact. But we wouldn't be able to produce as much of it as we're used to. This would mean a drop in the availability of beef, which would, like pork, have to become a special occasion food.

Prepared Foods

The following foods have been through some degree of processing, and they contain more than one ingredient. Many of them have local or homemade alternatives. For the remainder of the chapter, I'll throw in a little bit about alternative choices, where appropriate.

Prepared Foods: Small-Scale vs. Large-Scale Production

Food that's prepared in small batches is simply better than food produced on a mass scale. Ask any cook. This is especially so for these American favorites.

Small-Scale Production vs. Large-Scale Production: Cheese

Allow me to tell you a tale of two cheeses: industrially produced cream cheese—the kind produced by many large-scale food companies and sold in almost every grocery store—and the kind of artisanal soft cheese you might purchase from a small local dairy. With cheese, more than just about any other food, the two items are incomparable. They're not even meant to be consumed in the same way.

Taste. The taste of industrial cream cheese is decidedly monochromatic. It's the cheese equivalent of a breezy "Have a nice day!" uttered through a pasted-on smile. In contrast, the complexity of an artisanal cheese defies words. It's incomparable to *any* other food experience. You *do not* smear this glory on a sandwich or mix it into a recipe. The world stops turning while you're savoring this cheese.

Industrial cream cheese tastes about the same regardless of its point of purchase. For anyone with zero risk tolerance, this is comforting. But part of the fun of tasting local cheeses made in small batches is that you'll never taste two that are exactly the same. They inherit subtle differences from the environment in which the animals are pastured, the seasons, the climate, and the cheesemaking methods.

Economic impact. Artisanal cheese costs at least three times as much as industrial cheese, and that's as it should be. The real difference between these two cheeses is in the experience they create. The industrial product— convenient, cheap, and innocuous—is designed to be smeared on a bagel and eaten quickly while your mind is on other things. Artisanal cheese refuses to be eaten this way. It stops you in your tracks and demands your full attention.

Ultimately, it's meaningless to compare processed food from a supermarket with artisanal cheese from a small local producer because they aren't equivalent in any way, except that they both, inexplicably, bear the word "cheese." In fact, cheese itself, historically, was not eaten as an entrée but as a treat. You'd savor a few small slices before or after a meal, or with a glass of wine. Cheese has far too much fat and salt to make a healthy entrée.

When it comes to cheese, it's not just an issue of eating the same foods, only from local sources. It's a matter of changing our out-of-kilter foodways to ones that make more sense. Relegate cheese to the status of occasional treat, and you can afford the good stuff.

Convenience. Industrial cream cheese is available in almost any grocery store in the United States, and it's equally forgettable everywhere. Although you may have to look harder to find them and schedule a specific time to visit, small dairies and artisanal cheesemakers can be found in almost any part of the U.S., and nearly all of them can provide you with a unique and exquisite cheese experience. Good artisanal cheeses are also available at many upscale grocery stores, though they may not come from *local* cheesemakers.

Small-Scale vs. Large-Scale Production: Breakfast Cereal

Would you be willing to eat less of something delicious, if that smaller amount satisfied you more? Would you swap a little bit of convenience in exchange for a more meaningful eating experience? These are the kinds of questions that come into play when you compare store-bought granola with a cottage-made product you might find at a local farmers' market, co-op, or farm store. I can't answer these questions for you, but I can share my own experience with one particular cereal.

I discovered Bailey's Gems granola under a white awning at a farmers' market one sweltering day last July. I'm pretty sure the person I bought from was the company's owner. My kids ate it for breakfast the next morning and made me promise to go back and buy more of it the following week.

Convenience. While most supermarket chains offer several choices of industrially produced granola, to come by a bag of Bailey's Gems, I had to find the proprietor at a farmers' market. I can buy industrial granola on a whim 24/7, but I have to be serious enough about acquiring a cottage-made product to plan ahead.

Taste. To my sensibilities, store-bought granolas have the same overly sweet and otherwise-bland flavor of most processed foods. Bailey's Gems tastes like *real food*: the lemon peel in the Lemon Blueberry with Walnuts variety jumps right out.

Nutrition. Bailey's Gems Lemon Blueberry with Walnuts is made with real coconut flakes, lemon peel, dried blueberries, and walnuts. All the granola cereals at my local supermarket listed recognizable ingredients such as raisins, oats, and honey, but they also contained "natural flavors," those

Deadbeat Calories: Enriched White Flour

According to the USDA, when wheat is milled to make enriched white flour, twenty-five naturally occurring nutrients are removed, and five are replaced with chemical substitutes.

laboratory concoctions designed to help packaged supermarket foods regain some of the flavor lost to processing.

Economic impact. A ten-ounce brown paper zip-top bag of Bailey's Gems set me back $6.50 and provided about three bowls full of cereal. A 24-ounce box of store-bought granola runs between $4.50 and $4.99. That's a huge price difference for me, the consumer. But after the cash leaves my hands, the economics of the transaction are very different. Whenever I purchase a bag of Bailey's Gems cereal, 100 percent of the after-tax profits go to Bailey's Gems.

Environmental impact. The difference in environmental impact of these two foods can be attributed to their scales. Most of the brand-name granolas in my supermarket are owned by large food corporations, produced in one of several factories, and shipped long distances to grocery store shelves across the nation. All six of Bailey's Gems' products are made in her kitchen right here in my hometown. No additional infrastructure is required.

Substitution. By far the cheapest alternative to purchasing prepared granola is to buy the raw ingredients and assemble them at home. Combine rolled oats with just about any chopped nuts, fruits, and seeds you enjoy, plus a sweetener such as honey, agave, or syrup. Bake on low heat until lightly toasted. See the recipe for granola cereal on page 113.

Prepared Foods: Artificial vs. Natural Ingredients

Something happens to you when you begin to read food labels: you start to wonder what all that stuff really is, and what it's doing in your food. What does calcium propionate really add to your life, anyway? Certain supermarket foods have notoriously long lists of mysterious chemical ingredients. One of the worst offenders is bread, but the same could be said of almost any supermarket-bought baked good.

Artificial vs. Natural Ingredients: Tortillas

Sometimes, when I'm shopping with my family, I like to read the ingredients of packaged baked goods aloud. I'm serious—some of them are more scandalous than the checkout tabloids. "Aluminum phosphate? Fumaric acid? Sodium propionate? L-cysteine? Does this stuff sound *survivable*, let alone edible?" Doing this usually sends my kids scurrying to another aisle: *I don't know this lady. She just walked into the store with me.*

One day I scoured the big-chain grocery store nearest my house for baked items with fewer than six ingredients and came up empty-handed. Even the breads they made there at the store came loaded with a long list of unpronounceable ingredients. I gave up and began looking elsewhere.

I found Stacey's Organic Whole Wheat Flour Tortillas in my local food co-op. They're made in small batches through a Colorado-based cottage industry, and their flavor and texture are better than anything the grocery store can offer. Best of all, Stacey's tortillas contain exactly six ingredients, not counting water: whole-wheat flour, white flour, sunflower oil, baking powder, salt, and citric acid.

Convenience. While most large-chain supermarkets carry a selection of tortilla brands, Stacey's tortillas are available primarily at small organic specialty markets, which makes them slightly less convenient to purchase than their industrial counterparts.

Taste. Stacey's tortillas taste better than any other tortillas I've bought from a store.

Environment. Because Stacey's tortillas are sold in thirty-one states, according to her website, this rules them out as a *local* food choice in most of the places they're offered. The mileage aside, Stacy's tortillas leave a lighter footprint because making them involves less processing.

Artificial vs. Natural Ingredients: Sandwich Bread

The ingredients in most store-bought sandwich breads are so foreign to me that I can't determine whether or not they're food. Shortly after I gave up on grocery store bread, I discovered a small local bakery that produced a sandwich bread with only five ingredients, all of which I recognized. The Breadery, in Catonsville, Md., produces a 1.5-pound loaf of sandwich bread called Honey Whole Wheat. The Breadery's loaf contains only whole-wheat flour, water, honey, yeast, and salt.

Convenience. The Breadery's loaves are available at our local food co-op, but we get three loaves delivered with our milk each Friday from the local dairy that delivers our cheese, meat, and eggs. Because we order many other products from them, we pay no delivery fee, making this way of getting our bread far more convenient than schlepping to the store for it, and it also offsets much of the additional 96 cents we pay per loaf.

Taste. Because my kids are still in school, and still need portable lunches five days a week, it's presliced sandwich-sized loaves for us. Of this kind of bread, I think the Breadery's products taste the best. My husband and kids agree.

Nutrition. A slice of grocery-store bread contains about 4 percent of a person's daily calcium and iron. But the Breadery's slice also provides 8 percent thiamin, 5 percent niacin, 5 percent riboflavin, and 1 percent folate—nutrients that many store-bought breads don't list.

Economic impact. As of this writing, a loaf from the Breadery costs $4.95. The average loaf of store-bought bread runs anywhere between $1.99 and $5.99, plus the gas it costs to drive to the store for it.

Artificial vs. Natural Ingredients: Ice Cream

When it comes to this kid-classic food, it's the sheer number of industrial ingredients in supermarket ice creams that blows my mind. I've gone to several supermarket chains in search of ice cream that's made with just cream, sugar, salt, and vanilla. I've never found it.

Convenience. Real ice cream without all the added stuff is exceedingly rare in the supermarket world. You'll have to hunt around in natural food stores and co-ops, find a dairy that delivers it, or make it from scratch at home.

Taste. There's absolutely no comparison between the grocery store chemical concoction and fresh ice cream made from pure ingredients.

Substitution. Yes, you can make your own homemade ice cream! I've done it! This is another fun activity that absolutely blows kids' minds. You need fresh cream, sugar, vanilla extract, table salt, rock salt, crushed ice, and some sandwich-sized and some gallon-sized plastic zip bags. Combine cream, sugar, vanilla extract, and a pinch of table salt in a small bag, seal tight, and place it in a larger bag. Fill the large bag with ice and rock salt and seal it. Now, mush the bag around in as many creative ways as you can think of. Massage it, shake it, and hold it out while you do the Macarena. It takes a little while, but you'll eventually end up with homemade soft-serve vanilla ice cream!

Foods That Usually Can't Be Local

Up next are a few of the foods we Americans eat on a near-daily basis that, for most of us, simply can't be obtained locally. In the case of rice, coffee, tea, chocolate, sugar, and olive oil, these items come from tropical or semitropical plants that don't thrive in colder regions.

Foods That Usually Can't Be Local: Rice

Unlike wheat and corn, which are grown in most states, rice is a semitropical grain that isn't well suited to growing in most parts of the U.S. All fifty states can grow at least a little corn, forty-two states grow wheat, but only six states grow rice: Arkansas, California, Louisiana, Mississippi, Missouri, and Texas. To get truly local rice, by the strictest of definitions, you'd have to live in one of those states.

Economic impact. Growing rice requires a lot of labor. Historically, most rice has come from parts of the world where labor costs are low, which usually translates to low standards of living for those who work as rice growers.

Environmental impact. Rice farming typically requires a substantial and relatively permanent alteration of the landscape.

Substitution. If you want to keep most of your food purchases within a hundred-mile radius, and you're not close to a rice-growing state, try fresh local table corn, couscous, risoni, or other small rice-like wheat pastas.

Foods That Usually Can't Be Local: Coffee, Chocolate, Tea, and Sugar

If you're like me, you can barely imagine surviving without these four items. Unfortunately, they're a bit problematic from a local-organic-sustainable perspective, because they require a tropical or semitropical climate, something that most of the U.S. does not have. Alabama, Hawaii, Mississippi, Oregon, South Carolina, and Washington grow tea. Florida, Hawaii, Louisiana, and Texas grow sugar cane. Only Hawaii and, recently, California grow coffee beans for the commercial marketplace. Only Hawaii grows cocoa beans commercially.

Economic impact. If you buy these items imported, it's a good idea to check for the Fairtrade label on the package. Fair Trade certification on coffee, tea, sugar, fruits, or other farm products ensures that farm workers are paid a living wage and have access to health care, and that farmers can cover the cost of sustainable agriculture.

Substitution. Speaking strictly as an addict, as far as I'm concerned, there is no substitute for coffee, tea, and chocolate. Historically, chicory and certain grains have been ground and brewed as a coffee substitute whenever coffee supplies have run short, but none of these pack the wallop of caffeine that the real thing delivers. Likewise with chocolate and all cocoa-derived foods. Our family has found local honey to be a fine substitute for sugar in everything except baking, and we've felt better since we cut back on sugar.

Foods That Usually Can't Be Local: Olive Oil

This is the oil of choice for many Americans, because of its health benefits and rich flavor. At present, olive oil is produced commercially only in certain wine-growing regions of California, although some hobby farmers in other warm areas experiment with olive growing.

Substitution. The most local, and perhaps most sustainable, option is butter, since cattle can thrive in most parts of the United States. But butter's nutritional profile as a high-fat, high-cholesterol food makes it an iffy option. Canola oil is grown in certain regions of the U.S., has zero cholesterol, and can be used in the same way as olive oil.

I hope the information in this chapter has given you an example of some of the food choices that are out there. Some choices have a greater impact than others. Rather than gritting your teeth and becoming a purist—*I'm either 100 percent local-organic-all-the-time or I'm a failure*—what's doable is to try to make the best decisions we can with what's available and practical. Any given food decision may not be all at once the most nutritious, cost-effective, convenient, or environmentally sound, but overall, a long string of conscious, informed choices are bound to make a difference.

Granola Cereal

This recipe is *so easy*, and the flavor combinations are endless. I loved toasted hazelnut with dark chocolate chips. My family went ape over banana chips with coconut and almonds.

3 cups whole rolled oats

1 cup toasted chopped nuts (hazelnuts, almonds, peanuts, walnuts, pecans, macadamias)

1 cup dried fruit (raisins, sweetened coconut, banana chips, cranberries, blueberries)

1/2 cup seeds (sesame, flax, chia)

3/4 cup honey

1/4 cup oil

1 teaspoon spice (nutmeg, cinnamon)

optional: 1/2 cup dark chocolate chips

Preheat oven to 300 degrees. Combine dry ingredients, and then stir in honey and oil. (If you're adding chocolate chips, these must wait until the very end of the process, when the granola is completely cool.) Grease a baking pan, and spread granola evenly.

Bake for 10 to 15 minutes or until lightly toasted. Let cool thoroughly, then store in an airtight container. Keeps for about a week—or would, except if your kids are like mine they will eat up every last crumb of it the minute they find it. Make two batches. Hide the second.

7

Hunting and Gathering

Finding Sources of Local Food

Men are free when they belong to a living, organic, believing community. —*D. H. Lawrence*

I finished a bout of work late on a Saturday afternoon and drifted into the kitchen to find my three menfolk hard at work on dinner. My two sons were experimenting with a new technique they'd invented for flouring chicken wings for baking. It involved tossing the bag of flour, spices, and wings back and forth to each other like a football. They decided that, to make the chicken extra-tasty, they needed to do this tossing in every room in the house.

In the middle of the chaos, my husband worked like a sushi chef amid piles of chopped vegetables for his first-ever homemade coleslaw: shreds of cabbage the color of rubies, golden curls of carrot, and the mint-greens, sage-greens, and silver-greens of celery, kale, and shallots. The colors alone filled me with joy.

The making of a meaningful meal begins with the method of procurement. Most of our grocery store purchases get unceremoniously shoved into a corner of the fridge. That's just shopping, which is a chore. By contrast, this local stuff, grown with care and chosen with deliberation, deserves to be treated with a different kind of respect. I arrange pears, peppers, cabbages, and garlic in glass bowls with the same attention as cut flowers for the table. I open the fridge and I find works of art.

Preparing this food works all of my senses. Long before we taste it, there's the burst of colors; the ruffled, ruddy, earthen textures in my hands; the crinkle of leaves; and the peaty scent of soil that clings to them even after they're washed clean.

In this chapter, I'll describe ten different ways to obtain fresh local food. It's a good idea to cultivate as many local food sources as you can because, unlike the supermarket, where you can count on day-in, day-out sameness, local food is a little more mercurial than that. Prices vary, produce goes in and out of season, weather trends affect the quality of what's available, and local growers have different specialties. What one supplier can't do for you, another one might.

I've awarded each source one to five stars in two different categories: the sustainability of the methods by which their foods were produced and convenience to consumers. Five stars in a category means they're very sustainable or very convenient. One star means it may not be the most environmentally friendly option or it's not easy to fit into a busy suburban lifestyle. I've also awarded each source one to five dollar signs: one dollar indicates a comparatively inexpensive source; five dollars means it's pretty expensive. I'll round off the chapter with a few thoughts on how to integrate these sources to take advantage of the best that each has to offer.

Food Co-ops

Sustainability: ★ ★ ★ Convenience: ★ ★ ★ ★ ★ Price: $$$$$

Quite possibly the most convenient way to buy local-organic-sustainable produce is through your local food co-op: an organization of enthusiastic employees and volunteers dedicated to bringing great food to their community. Co-ops run the gamut from small sandwich counters with a few bins of organic produce to ultramodern supermarket-inspired venues that carry almost everything a grocery store might. Food co-ops rose to popularity in the 1960s and 1970s and, in subtle ways, many of them retain some of the culture of those times.

Food co-ops are the perfect first step in your transition from supermarket food to organic, sustainable, and local options because, compared with most of the choices you'll find in this chapter, they're more similar to the supermarket experience. If you'd prefer to wean yourself off the grocery store slowly, co-ops are a good way to go.

Shopping at our local food co-op feels like a treat, an outing, not a chore. Rather than the harried, stressed, and depleted sensation that accompanies supermarket shopping, when I come out of the co-op, I feel as though we've done something fun, benevolent, and good for us, all in one stop. The "fun" part comes from the relaxed and friendly vibe the place and its staff exudes.

The "good for us" part resides in the food choices, most of them organic, many of them local, and some of them cooked there on the spot. The feeling of benevolence is generated by the bins at the exit that collect donations for local charities.

A co-op by definition is an association of people who join together to meet common economic and social needs, which they do through a jointly owned, democratically managed business model.

Just so you know, not everything in a given co-op is guaranteed to be local, organic, or even sustainable. Unless they specialize in offering exclusively local food, you may find offerings from the industrial food system on their shelves, and you may discover that a lot of their organic produce comes from California, especially in the winter. But overall, the emphasis in food co-ops is on quality and health, and many of them will opt for local foods as often as they can get them. If you're trying to be a purist, and you want to eliminate *all* industrial foods from your diet, you'd probably have to shop with caution at your local co-op. But if you're happy with *mostly* organic-sustainable choices, a co-op will fill your grocery bags nicely.

Are co-ops more expensive than large chain supermarkets? As a general rule, yes. They typically run 20 to 30 percent more than the cost of roughly comparable items at the grocery store, simply because the economic law of supply and demand dictates that smaller-scale production must be priced higher than mass production. This, and the cost of staffing and maintaining a physical location, makes the food co-op one of the priciest options in this chapter. But it may make up for this higher cost with greater convenience. Your local co-op will probably stay open year-round, long after your favorite farmers' market is buttoned down tight for the winter. Plus, you're more likely to manage one-stop shopping here than from most other local sources.

How can you make the cost of a co-op more affordable? If you avail yourself of the cheaper choices, such as farmers' markets, during the parts of the year they're open, you will probably find that you can offset the higher cost of shopping at the co-op during winter months. Also, many co-ops offer a membership or ownership program, which, for an upfront fee, entitles you to certain discounts and can help lower the cost. Some co-ops, but not all, require their members to work a certain number of hours as part of their membership responsibilities. The details of any such requirements will be spelled out in their membership application.

The Common Market Food Co-op: Corporation With a Conscience

If you're used to the sterile anonymity of big-chain supermarkets, brace yourself for a paradigm shift. From the moment you step into your local food co-op, you'll notice the difference. For my family, discovering the Common Market in Frederick, Md., was one of the first experiences that launched us on our local-sustainable food journey. Shopping there has been one of the key ways we've kept ourselves engaged in a meaningful food life.

Recently, I asked Marketing Manager Sally Fulmer and Education Specialist Zoe Brittain to tell me what they love most about working at the Common Market.

Zoe told me her job is all about "making the world a better place in which to live, eat, and do business. It's the two-way exchange of ideas and inspiration that really gets me going."

Sally gave me an example of the Common Market's worldview in action: "We take into consideration environmental and social concerns. We don't just base our decisions on maximizing profit. We educate our shoppers so they can make informed decisions about their food choices." She spoke of "transparency" in the same vein I've heard from local farmers. "We only carry products that our owners and shoppers request and that fit our buying standards. We never accept money from vendors or manufacturers in exchange for carrying their products."

Unlike your local big-chain supermarket, you can actually sign up to own a piece of the Common Market. Sally explained that co-op ownership gives members "a democratic say in how the business is run and an influence on the direction of our future."

The Common Market carries items from more than forty-five local farms and fifty-eight local businesses. It's the common ground between co-op and producer, not the bottom line, that guides their decision to carry an item. "We look for shared values and priorities," Zoe told me. "If it seems like a product would fit, our buyers will meet with the producer and find out what makes the product special."

Because cost seems to be the biggest concern for the would-be-local shoppers I've talked to, I asked Zoe how she explains the price difference to their customers. "I try to introduce the idea of the true cost of food," Zoe explained. "When food is priced low, someone or something else is paying the price instead of the consumer."

One of my favorite parts of shopping at the co-op comes at the end, when we get a poker chip for each paper bag we bring in to reuse. At the exit, we can choose among four charities to "invest" our chips. The Common Market donates ten cents for each chip that customers place in a charity's basket. Zoe told me that since they implemented the Bring-a-Bag poker chip system, they've raised $86,000 for local nonprofits and saved 784,000 bags from the landfill. How do they decide which charities will benefit from the chips? "We choose four nonprofits each quarter, one each to represent environmental, social, animal, and child well-being."

So, what's the bottom-line difference between a food co-op and a big-chain supermarket? Shopping at the Common Market is never just about buying groceries. It's a chance to savor great food, connect with the community, and enjoy the satisfaction of shopping in harmony with our worldview.

Rock Stars and Local Farmers: No One Beats Their Popularity

Who could have predicted the stellar rise in popularity that local farmers have enjoyed over the past few years? We're talking megatrend here. And it's largely because Americans have *finally* discovered farmers' markets. The number of markets in the United States has increased 26 percent since the mid 1990s. As of 2013, Americans could visit a whopping 8,144 farmers' markets. Local farmers are *hot!*

If you'd like to find a co-op near you, visit the Coop Directory Service at www.coopdirectory.org.

Farmers' Markets

Sustainability: ★★★★★ Convenience: ★★ Price: $$

Our first trip to a farmers' market on a sunny Saturday morning felt more like a vacation than a grocery-shopping trip. The scene that unfolded before us could have been some sort of festival: white canvas awnings flapping in a warm breeze. Sprays of hollyhocks and sunflowers. A carnival of shining peppers, every color of the rainbow, spilling out of bushel baskets. Goat cheeses, homemade cinnamon loaves, cider. Hand-dyed, homespun wool. Free samples. Brisk trade. Dogs and kids. Happy conversation. We went home with two loaves of crusty bread, a bag bursting with ripe tomatoes, and four smiles.

We're living in a wondrous era in which the number of farmers' markets nationwide is booming. They've made their way into many urban and suburban areas, bringing the bounty of the farm to the people.

Farmers' markets are comparable in price to supermarkets, and often much cheaper, depending on what you're after, but there's no comparison when it comes to quality. The food at the farmers' market is much fresher than grocery store fare. You're usually buying it directly from the people who grew it, so you can talk to them about it. Best of all, once you get the hang of buying seasonally, you can ask them, "What do you have a lot of that you'd like to unload?" It's win-win: you'll be doing them a favor, as well as yourself. You can take home the bounty you scored and freeze it. Doing this can go a long way toward offsetting the higher upfront cost of local-organic-sustainable food.

Farmers' markets pop up in an array of locations, from office parking lots that are empty for the weekend to parks, fairgrounds, and the grassy lawns in front of public buildings.

To make the most use of a farmers' market, plan to take advantage of whatever's on offer, rather than coming with a set of expectations. Because the availability of any given local food is driven by the seasonality of crops, they're not guaranteed to have what you're after. They have what they have. If you came in looking for radicchio but go home with snow leopard melons, that's part of the adventure.

Hometown Harvest: Farmers' Market on Your Doorstep

Baltimore, Md., Summer 2009: one sweltering Saturday morning, farmer Tony Brusco manned his produce stand at a bustling downtown farmers' market. Although he loved the market itself, he began to wonder if the crowds and horrendous parking might be driving some customers away. He talked it over with his fellow farmers, and then with customers. "What I found was that folks wanted to buy local, but the traditional channels weren't as convenient as they once were," he said.

Tony decided to create a business that would bring farmers' market produce straight to the consumer's door: "I figured I would make the deliveries from the back of my pickup truck with my kids as a way of providing a service, while also teaching them something about business." He thought a website would be the most convenient way for busy shoppers to order, though he admits, "I still wasn't confident that people would shop at a farmers' market online."

That summer, Tony and his wife, Abby, launched Hometown Harvest from their home in Middletown, Md. For the first few months, they managed the business part-time, making between 100 and 150 deliveries a week. "Eventually, around Christmastime, we felt that we had enough business that we could carefully step away from our regular jobs and do this full-time." Since then, they've built a devoted staff of people who are passionate about fresh food.

Tony told me that what he likes about Hometown Harvest's business model is that it provides services to both their customers and their farmers: "We offer customers a convenient way to buy local, and because we work with so many farmers, we offer a wide variety of items. We give farmers access to customers they wouldn't otherwise be able to sell to. We basically offer them a farmers' market, but they don't have to staff it or spend hours away from their farms." Hometown Harvest also does exhaustive research on their farmers and producers, ensuring that everything customers purchase from them meets a high standard and verifying producers' claims. "If we say the eggs are from pastured chickens, we've personally been to that farm and seen the chickens out on pasture," he said.

After doing a little research and finding Hometown Harvest on the USDA's Working List of Food Hubs, I asked Tony what the proper name was for the kind of service his company provides. He replied, "I have honestly never spent a lot of time looking for an official name for what we do. I simply describe our service as an online farmers' market that comes to you."

Tony supports the consumer's right to be informed about the way produce is grown and animals are handled. He feels it's important for people to know and trust where their food is coming from because, as he puts it, "food is the fuel of life."

Shopping at a farmers' market usually means carrying your own bags. Some vendors have them, and others don't. Likewise with cash: larger operations may take credit cards, but old-fashioned paper bills and coins are still accepted at every booth.

The main drawback to farmers' markets, at least from the perspective of us suburban convenience-hounds, is that they operate for a limited set of hours. Saturday mornings are the usual times, and maybe Sundays. Some, but not many, farmers' markets meet on weekday afternoons. Except in the southernmost regions of the country, they're almost all seasonal: few of them open before May, and not many will linger past October. In Chapter 10, I'll talk about some of the ways we learned to manage our winter farmers'-market-withdrawal symptoms.

To find farmers' markets in your area, visit www.localharvest.org. You can also visit your town's website and search "farmers' markets."

Direct From the Farm

Sustainability: ★ ★ ★ ★ Convenience: ★ Price: $$

Nothing quite beats driving out to your local farm, taking in the ambience, meeting the people who grow your sustenance, and buying from them directly. This is the purest of all local food encounters, unless you count growing it yourself. You'll learn more, open yourself more, and come away more transformed than with any other local food-buying method. If you find a local farm that offers a pick-your-own-produce experience, you've struck gold.

What you don't want to do, though, is show up unannounced, outside the farm's regularly scheduled public hours. Farms that sell directly to the public usually establish specific days and times for doing so. Otherwise, they may ask you to call ahead to schedule a time to visit. Check your farm's website for their public selling hours, or call to ask for an appointment.

On a similar note, many farms advertise that they're completely open to the public, and many even encourage you to take a self-guided tour. If they say this is okay, by all means, don't miss out on a chance to explore and learn, but be careful not to get in the way of anyone's work. Stay out of planted fields and animal enclosures. Keep away from machinery. Stay well clear of private residences. Don't enter buildings unless you see signs expressly permitting you to enter.

A word to the wise: whatever you do, don't complain about what you see! We suburban folk tend to be a bit on the ethnocentric side. We judge life on the farm by the standards of our own lives. At Nick Maravell's Organic Farm in Adamstown, Md., a large red and white sign on the sales barn warns visitors of these differences: farms don't smell quite the same as your living room, feral barn cats aren't as approachable as house cats, and farm animals like to have sex outdoors, even in front of impressionable small children. If, while visiting a farm, you see, smell, or hear something that offends or boggles you, stay in polite visitor mode and keep yourself in a learning frame of mind!

To find farms in your area, check out your city's website and search "farms" or "agriculture." You may find that your area sponsors one or two annual open house days at local farms. One weekend every October, many farms in our area throw open their doors and offer food tastings, crafts for kids, hayrides, and opportunities to pet the animals. Events such as these are marvelous opportunities to engage the family in farm life.

CSAs

Sustainability: ★ ★ ★ ★ ★ Convenience: ★ ★ ★ Price: $$$$$

CSA stands for "Community Supported Agriculture." In other words, you, as a member of the farmer's community, pay him directly for growing food for you. This idea is a smart solution to an age-old cash-flow issue: farmers needed the biggest chunk of capital in the spring—for seeds, fertilizer, equipment, and labor—to get crops into the ground. This just happens to be the time when most farmers are cash-poor, after a long winter with no crops. Someone got the bright idea that if we eaters could put up a chunk of cash in the spring, farmers could then feed us on a regular basis throughout the growing season.

The classic arrangement for a CSA involves signing up in early spring and paying a few hundred dollars upfront. Then, as the harvests begin to roll in, you collect a box of whatever's in season, usually once a week from May to October. Typically, you drive to the farm to pick up your box, but as CSAs have become more popular, some farms have begun to offer a delivery service. For an extra fee, your freshly picked farm goodies come right to your door. The other nice development that's come along, since people have

Open Book Farm: A Tale of Sustainable Growing

One of the greatest pleasures of eating locally is the opportunity to visit the place where your food is grown. One of the first farms we visited, when we were just beginning to fall in love with local food, was Open Book Farm in Myersville, Md., a small, diversified livestock and vegetable farm run by Mary Kathryn and Andrew Barnet. Even the name they chose for their farm conveys the commitment to transparency and the welcoming attitude for which small-scale farmers are known.

We visited Open Book Farm one brisk October afternoon. The first member of the Barnet family to greet us was Patou, the friendly Great Pyrenees dog, whose job it is to guard the chickens and turkeys. Next, Mary Kathryn Barnet emerged from the farmhouse, introduced herself, and took us on a guided tour of the farm.

M. K. brought us into her greenhouses where flats of spinach sprouted and red bell peppers glowed on the vine. She took us to the barn where her customers stuff their CSA bags each weekend of the growing season with their pick of produce. Then she walked us out to the emerald field where she kept her chickens: five mobile enclosures, each full of lively birds, lined up in neat rows. They looked like they were mowing her lawn for her, the way a bunch of neighborhood kids might have done. I half expected they'd hit her up for a twenty when they got to the end of the rows.

The pigs had already gone to market for that season, but M. K. showed us the fine work their hooves and rooting snouts had done to enliven the soil. Noticing the absence of tilled crops, other than those inside the greenhouse and in one small garden, I later asked her if Open Book counted as a grass farm.

"The livestock part of the farm is absolutely a grass farm," she replied. "The livestock and the vegetables benefit each other." She and Andrew had started with chickens, pigs, and turkeys because they were small, took only one season to raise, and were relatively easy to market, but Andrew's real passion has always been beef cattle, which they started raising in the spring of 2014. "Cows are so good for the land," M. K. explained. "They live entirely on grass."

I asked how they came up with the idea of a winter CSA, currently the only one of its kind in the area. "We started in July, so we didn't have time to grow summer vegetables," she replied. They decided to grow fall vegetables in time to offer their first winter CSA. "Because a winter CSA was so unusual, the *Frederick News Post* did a story on us," she said, and from that day forward, their popularity began to grow.

From the abundance and order of the place, I'd have thought this farm had been around for decades, and that Andrew and Mary Kathryn had been born to farming. I was surprised when she later told me "we're both city kids" and went on to explain that Open Book Farm was less than three years old. She came to farming after completing a degree in international development, which led her to an interest in sustainable agriculture.

To this day, she's passionate about making great food available to people. "Everybody needs it," she told me, "and everybody needs it to be wholesome and nourishing." Her husband, Andrew, she explained, was drawn to farming because he wanted to see the "cause and effect" of good agricultural practices and their influence on the land.

In this vibrant place, the effect of their loving stewardship is written across these lush green acres like words on the pages of a storybook.

been discovering CSAs, is that some of them now offer the ability to pay on a month-to-month basis, rather than requiring that you come up with a large sum at the beginning of the season.

What will you find in your CSA box when you go to pick it up? That's the fun part, or the frustrating part, depending on how comfortable you are with surprises. Your CSA farmer will give you a mix of whatever he's got. A colleague of mine who invested in a CSA recalls a time in mid June when practically all her farmer had ready was his crop of basil: for about three weeks in a row, she found her box stuffed with bunches of aromatic basil leaves, and little else. She had almost run out of places to stash quarts of homemade pesto before the first tomatoes and peppers finally began to show up in place of the herbs.

Some farms are able to offer their customers a certain amount of choice in the contents of their weekly share. At Open Book Farm (see the sidebar), CSA subscribers stuff their own bags in a large, airy former milk barn. Open Book's summer CSA is a "free choice volume share": customers can fill their bags with as much as they want of the veggies they love and opt out of the ones they don't.

Most farms offer spring, summer, and fall CSA subscriptions, but few provide a winter CSA plan. For around $400, Open Book Farm provides subscribers with a "winter storage share": once a month, roughly November through February, customers drive to the milk barn to pick up their portion of frozen pastured meats; eggs; stockpiled items such as onions, apples, cabbage, potatoes, garlic, and squashes; and fresh fare such as carrots, beets, spinach, lettuce, arugula, sweet turnips, bok choi, collards, and leeks from the farm's two greenhouses.

For busy working folks, CSAs are a great approach to keeping the family supplied with local produce. But the cost of a CSA can prove a bit daunting. There's a reason why a CSA ends up being more costly than simply buying a random bag full of produce from a local farmer: to the price of the food, CSAs must add the costs they incur for packing materials and labor hours from managing CSA subscriptions and packing the items.

To find CSAs in your area, visit www.localharvest.org, where you can plug in your zip code or state and see a list of farms near you that offer CSA subscriptions.

Top Nine Places to Avoid Getting Your Food, If You're Trying to Eat Fresh and Local

1. Prisons
2. School cafeterias
3. Military mess halls
4. Fast food restaurants
5. Gas stations
6. Convenience stores
7. Vending machines
8. Snack bars
9. Amusement parks

Buying Clubs

Sustainability: ★ ★ ★ ★ Convenience: ★ ★ ★ ★ Price: $$$

This is a particularly nice option for folks who live in or near large urban areas. With buying clubs, customers band together and use their combined buying power to purchase large quantities of fresh farm produce for less than what it would cost each family to purchase the same items in small quantities. Their purchase is then delivered for pickup at a central location at a regularly scheduled date and time.

Although this system hits a home run when it comes to convenience, it misses the mark a little in terms of the overall farm experience. It doesn't put you onto farmland or in direct communication with farmers. You won't get to pet any pigs or pick any cherries this way. And it doesn't offer you the chance to browse, peruse, explore, or experiment with a new food you just happen upon, because what shows up at the distribution point is supposed to be just what you ordered. It's a more utilitarian—in other words, not as fun—way to access local food. But it does save a lot of time and still ensures that your food bucks go to farmers in your area.

To tap into a buyer's network near you, visit www.localharvest.org or browse your favorite farmers' websites and see if any of them offer a buyer's club option. If they don't, you could always chat about it with some friends and neighbors and see if they might want to start one with you.

Supermarket

Sustainability: ★ Convenience: ★ ★ ★ ★ ★ Price: $$$

When you make the commitment to eating most of your food from local sources, you probably won't quit your local supermarket cold turkey. You'll still drop in from time to time for the things you can't get from the goat dairy down the road or the apple orchard just outside of town.

This morning, I visited the grocery store where we used to do almost all of our shopping. They hadn't even seen me since the previous month, not that they noticed. Until about a year ago, had anyone at the store actually been paying attention to us, they would have seen our family arrive late each Sunday morning and fill two carts with everything from pizza bites to frozen waffles. We don't eat like that anymore. Today, my cart contained laundry detergent, deodorant, and cat food—items I'd never expect to see for sale at my local farm. Because we sometimes need items like these, I'm grateful the supermarket is still there for me, although our relationship, if you can call it that, has changed a bit.

Supermarkets are great for nonfood necessities. They're also the most convenient go-to place if you forgot to buy sandwich bread for school lunches and you don't remember until 10:30 at night, your son says he absolutely can't make sausage noodles for tonight's dinner without an onion, or the biscuit recipe calls for cream of tartar and you're not even sure what that is, let alone what kind of local farmer would grow it. I've gradually learned that these situations are not really the national crises they seem to be at the time, but it's awfully nice to have a solution for them in the form of the supermarket, five minutes away, that's never, ever closed for the season.

If, for whatever reason, you find yourself in a circumstance in which you do have to buy the bulk of your groceries from a supermarket, there are ways to make it a healthier, more sustainable trip. First, shop as much as you can on the periphery of the store and steer clear of the aisles. The food you'll find up against the store walls is the fresher stuff: items that need to be refrigerated, chilled, or sprayed with water. The food on the shelves in the aisles is the practically indestructible processed stuff wrapped in layers of plastic, with packaging bearing long lists of ingredients that an English professor would have trouble pronouncing.

Can you find organic foods at your local supermarket? You might. Many grocery store chains have been steadily expanding their selections of organics in response to consumer demand. If you do have to buy nonorganic produce, choose the ones with inedible skins such as bananas, oranges, and avocados. The skin makes something of a barrier between you and the pesticides with which they've been sprayed. Try to avoid nonorganic leaves such as spinach, lettuce, and kale, and all animal products, because these are almost certainly from CAFOs. Buy the simplest ingredients you can: flour, salt, and baking powder, rather than biscuit mix. This saves you money and cuts down on the amount of processing the food has had to endure.

What about locally grown foods? Can any of these be found in the big-chain grocery stores? As of this writing, local farmers are woefully underrepresented at supermarkets in my area. If you're incredibly lucky, you might find a few offerings of local fruits and vegetables in their produce sections. Supermarket chains prefer to buy in bulk: large, uniform ship-ments that arrive on a regular basis. This is what the industrial food system supplies them. The small, seasonal offerings of local producers don't fit their business models. But as the demand for local produce rises, this may change.

Big-Chain Organic Markets

Sustainability: ★ ★ Convenience: ★ ★ ★ ★ Price: $$$$$

Large industrial supermarket chains that specialize in organics are yet another resource for organic and sustainable foods, but not everything they carry will automatically fit the criteria you have in mind. Some will be organic processed food, in which the various food components were grown organically before they were processed and assembled in a factory. It's not the devil, but it's not the same thing as buying whole fresh foods from local growers. Processed organics do little to enhance the socioeconomic health of communities or to reduce the amount of fossil fuel burned to move food from processing plants to warehouses to points-of-purchase.

Having said this, I've also found that big-chain organic stores in my area do make an effort to stock a certain amount of locally produced foods. As I browse the produce aisles and refrigerator cases, I can find meats, cheeses, fruits, and vegetables from local farms whose names I know. Often, when the food is local, the store will prominently display its source on signage close to the item. Best of all, one chain I visited recently advertises the CSAs for the local farms whose produce they carry.

The best time to patronize large organic chain stores is when you're af-ter some kind of specialty item, something you're pretty sure your farmers' market is not going to carry. They're also a reasonable option for feeding yourself on organic produce during winter months, when most of your local suppliers will be settled in for a long nap. Most of the fruits and vegetables on offer probably won't be local, but you may choose to relax the hundred-mile rule in favor of being able to keep your family supplied with fresh organic produce through the winter.

Your Backyard

Sustainability: ★ ★ ★ ★ ★   Convenience: ★   Price: $

Now we're really talking local! For environmental sustainability, lowest cost, freshest flavor, and sheer connection to the web of life, nothing beats the food you grow at home. If you can grow anything at all, even if it's just a patio planter full of five-color chard, don't miss out on this experience. Because it's the purest way to feed yourself, because it harmonizes so beautifully with the principles I'm laying out in this book, and because it's one of the most rewarding things you can possibly do with your time, I've devoted the whole of Chapter 11 to the most local of all food sources, your backyard.

Your Neighbor's Backyard

Sustainability: ★ ★ ★ ★ ★   Convenience: ★   Price: $

The way I titled this section, I make it sound like I'm advocating sneaking out in the middle of the night and filching from your neighbor's pepper patch. What I mean to imply here is that if you grow a little food in your backyard, and your neighbor does too, you could set up an exchange.

Odds are, she's not going to grow exactly the same things you do. In late July, of course, you'll be trying to bury each other in tomatoes and zucchinis, because that's what every backyard gardener is doing. But for most of the growing season, you can swap your specialty for what she grows best.

There's no reason why the exchange has to be limited to garden produce. If she gardens and you have a gray thumb, you can exchange whatever you've got that she needs: editing, piano lessons, dog walking. This form of economic exchange, known among anthropologists as reciprocity, is as old as humankind itself, was the only kind of economic system we had for the first two million years of human existence, and in certain important ways, has never been improved upon.

Your Community Garden

Sustainability: ★ ★ ★ ★ ★   Convenience: ★   Price: $

There's one more marvelous way to avail yourself of fresh locally grown produce: by joining a local community garden. Community gardens are

What About Local Vino? Five States That Produce Wine

California
Maryland
Oregon
Virginia
Washington

Which Sources Fit Your Priorities?

If Your Priority Is...	...Try These Sources
Convenience	Food co-ops, delivery service, organic supermarkets
Buying only from local growers	Direct from farm, CSAs, farmer's markets
Sustainability	Grow your own, community garden, direct from farm
Low cost	Grow your own, community garden, direct from farm
Animal welfare	Grow your own, direct from farm
Community connections	Food co-ops, community garden, farmer's markets
Fun	Direct from farm, farmer's markets, community garden

built, maintained, and shared collectively by members of a neighborhood. Some community gardens are informal. Others are managed through an association. A community garden provides a wonderful social outlet as well as nutritious, delicious local food. It also minimizes gardening effort, time, and cost by pooling neighborhood resources. Find a community garden near you by visiting the American Community Gardening Association's website at www.communitygarden.org and entering your zip code.

Putting It All Together

To avail yourself of the best possible options in price, selection, community, sustainability, and convenience, the best strategy is to cultivate several of these sources. That's the most fun way to do it, because it puts you in contact with the broadest range of people and experiences.

You can combine the lowest cost with the most fun by visiting farms and farmers' markets whenever you can, and stopping at a co-op or organic market on the way home for anything you couldn't get during your outing. Sign up for CSAs and delivery services for the things you use on a regular basis. This strategy will probably only work for you during the growing season, unless you can find enough farms that operate year-round.

If you're an avid vegetable gardener, you may not need a CSA share for part of the growing season because you're functioning as your own CSA. One gardener I know purchases a spring and fall CSA share from a local farm, but not a summer share, because in June, July, and August, she's wading through her own avalanche of homegrown produce.

If you prefer the more mainstream feel of shopping at a co-op or organic supermarket, but you'd like to offset the cost a little, try buying most of your groceries at these places, but ordering your meats, eggs, and dairy from a local source that offers delivery. Food from any storefront-type operation is going to be more expensive because they have to mark up their products to cover the cost of their overhead. This price boost shows up the largest on higher-ticket items, which in most cases means meat. If you get the pricier stuff directly from the grower and use the store for the rest, you'll strike a balance between cost and convenience.

I'll tell you a little bit about how we have combined some of these options, so you can get an idea of how it can work for a busy family. Once or twice a month, we make a regular grocery trip to our local food co-op, for pasta, rice, canned tomatoes, and bakery items, but during the growing season, it's the *last* stop on the grocery-procurement tour, not because we don't love shopping there, but because they're the most expensive option. We go to them last because they're certain to have the items we can't find at our other sources.

Year-round, once a week, we automatically order our milk and some of our meat from a local dairy that delivers, mostly because my husband, Al, is addicted to their creamy grass-fed milk in glass bottles. The delivery arrives on our carport before 5:00 a.m. every Friday morning. When we're not up to our eyeballs in fresh vegetables from our own garden, we get a weekly bag of assorted whatever's-in-season from Hometown Harvest, which arrives on the carport on Tuesdays. A pair of large coolers maintain permanent residence on our carport for these deliveries.

During the growing season, which in our region is roughly May to October, we've shopped at two local farmers' markets: a large one that operates on Saturdays and a smaller one that opens for a few hours each Tuesday afternoon.

In addition to these sources, we've made a habit of taking afternoon trips to local farms about once a month, just because we love them. Wherever we end up, we meet the farmers, enjoy the fresh air, pet the animals, and buy a little bit of whatever they have to offer. Do we still visit the rank-and-file grocery stores? Yes, but only to fill in what we can't get from these other sources.

We've fallen into a nice routine that gives us the right combo of low price, convenience, and a sense of adventure. Ours is tailor-made for us. One of the joys you have to look forward to is developing your own local-food-foraging itinerary.

Moose Wings

My son Phillip, aka Moose, devised this recipe. It can be made entirely with local ingredients with the exception of the paprika, chipotle, and chili powders.

12–16 chicken wings

1 cup milk

1 beaten egg

1 cup flour

1 teaspoon salt

2 teaspoons chili powder

1/2 teaspoon paprika

1/2 teaspoon chipotle powder

1 cup toasted bread crumbs

Beat the eggs and add milk. Soak chicken wings in the milk and egg mixture for five minutes. Place all dry ingredients in a plastic bag and shake. Drop chicken wings two or three at a time into the plastic bag and shake in every room in the house, or until coated.

Arrange the wings on a baking tray. Bake at 400 degrees until crispy brown and fully cooked (about 30 minutes).

8

It Can Be Done

How to Make Local, Organic, and Sustainable Food Cost Less Than Supermarket Food

The price of anything is the amount of life you exchange for it. —*Henry David Thoreau*

Here it is—the chapter that stretches my credibility the most.

You've probably heard it so many times by now that you wouldn't dream of questioning it: local, organic, sustainably produced food is *way* more expensive than regular food. It's just a gimmick. It's for food snobs. You can't afford it. It's not for you.

Every news story I've encountered, in print and on TV, promotes this line of thinking. I've never seen even one article offering tips on how to reduce the cost of these foods. This is why I set myself the task of proving that it could be done.

Over the past two years, as my obsession with alternative food choices grew, my family has gamely switched from a diet based largely on processed supermarket food to one that comes mostly from local farms, many of which are organic. At first, this switch was certainly *not* cheaper. Initially, our weekly grocery bill rose by 20 to 30 percent. To offset this additional expense, we quit eating out at restaurants for a while and, that first summer, we took our family vacation in a tent at a state park instead of a hotel at the beach. But as we spent a few more seasons experimenting with the options, we began to get the hang of it. Then, slowly and surely, our weekly outlay for groceries began to drop. Most weeks, it now hovers between the same amount it was during our supermarket days and, depending on the season, 10 to 20 percent *less.*

Of course, there's one simple principle to eating local-organic-sustainable food for less than you pay at the supermarket: you'll have to change *what* you're eating. You absolutely could not buy all of the same foods you've been getting at the grocery store, in a local-organic-sustainable form, and pay less for them. To make local food cost less takes change in many directions: the kinds of foods you choose, the time of year you buy them, the quantities you buy, the way you prepare them, and much more.

In this chapter, I'll explain why the price is higher for local foods, and why that's fair. I'll compare the cost of local food sources with that of grocery stores in terms of the percentage of your overall grocery budget. Then we'll talk about how to mix and match sources to get the best prices. After that, I'll share some other rules of thumb that will help reduce the cost of great local food.

Why Local Food Is Usually More Expensive— and Should Be

We supermarket foragers have come to expect our groceries to be cheap. We tend to react with outrage whenever we see a higher price tag on an everyday food item. But we only think this way because industrially produced food has become *normal* for us. We forget that mass-produced food is a historical anomaly.

The impetus behind the local food movement, and behind the writing of this book, is that what seems cheap and convenient on the surface has hidden costs, deferred expenses, and a high price to be paid in many other aspects of our lives.

The true cost of a thing doesn't go away just because its price is cheap.

In reality, food production has *always* had a high cost. That's why our hunter-gatherer ancestors only made the switch from foraging out of sheer necessity. Many of the methods the industrial food system relies on today were first invented in an attempt to deploy the "faster-cheaper-more" efficiency of the factory assembly line to food production. Unfortunately, it didn't lower the *ultimate* cost, only the immediate, upfront cost. As we're finding out now, we will still have to pay the piper.

Often, we suburban consumers aren't aware of the true costs involved in small-scale food production. The costs for taxes, labor, fuel, quality assurance, and insurance take a deeper bite out of a small farmer's profit margin than they do out of large-scale producers'. Many small-scale farmers feel that it's important to get to know their customers and answer their questions. This is part of what they mean by "transparency of method." But farmers receive no monetary recompense for the time it takes to make themselves available.

Another factor that drives up the price of local food is the cost of complying with federal food safety mandates. Large-scale producers find it easier to command the kinds of profits it takes to invest in the infrastructure and labor costs necessary to achieve compliance. The real irony is that the major outbreaks of food-borne illnesses that have prompted new safety legislation have seldom been linked to small-scale producers.

In a November 2013 *Huffington Post* article, columnist Jim Slama wrote that the FDA is preparing new regulations aimed at preventing food contamination. Unfortunately, the prevention methods they propose will be costly. According to Slama, the way the math works out with these new regulations, farms that net less than $500,000 in sales will end up paying "4 to 6 percent of their gross revenues to comply." Many small farmers, who already operate on a narrow profit margin, may find that this is too large a hit for them to take and still remain afloat.

This added burden comes at a time when the federal government seems to be withdrawing support for small local producers. Slama points out that Congress did not renew funding for most of the programs designed to support small farmers, even though they make up "the fastest growing section of the food economy."

A third factor that drives up the cost of local food production falls under the heading of consumer expectations. Customers sometimes arrive at farm stores and roadside stands thinking the produce there will be identical to what the supermarket has on offer. Many suburban consumers have little idea that the waxy perfection and uniformity of grocery store produce is a highly artificial contrivance. Some customers expect a small farm store to offer the same selections as the supermarket, and to have the same amounts of their favorites on hand regardless of season.

When we buy from local farmers, we need to keep in mind that they feel the effects of high production costs much more than large-scale producers do, and they can seldom access the same government subsidies to offset those expenses. They're expected to meet government standards that are usually designed with large-scale producers in mind, and they must do it with a dwindling amount of support. We need to understand that a small, family-run operation is not going to offer the breadth of variety we're

It's Not Apples to Apples

When I asked organic farmer Nick Maravell to comment on the price of local food, he replied, "In reality, some organic food costs more. There are additional costs involved in becoming certified organic. But a lot of organic food is competitively priced. It depends on where and how you buy it." He explained that the law of supply and demand influences the price as well: "People pay more because there's less supply." Rather than comparing prices, Nick wants consumers to understand that local, organic food is not comparable to supermarket food. "In many cases, you won't find that product in the grocery store," he said.

accustomed to, and that they are subject to the limitations of seasonality. They work long days, often short-handed. They battle the uncertainties of weather, pests, and crop diseases with little government assistance, and at the end of the harvest, they sometimes face exacting customers with long lists of demands.

If we want to reduce the cost of food, it should not be at their expense. If we're willing to pay the true price of the good food they grow for us, we can still reduce our overall food expenses by being smarter consumers.

Local Sources: A Side-by-Side Cost Comparison

In this section, I'll compare the overall cost of obtaining food from co-ops, farmers' markets, CSAs, directly from farmers, and growing your own with the cost of procuring the same *amount* of food at big-chain supermarkets. By amount, I'm referring primarily to the number of calories it takes to feed a family of four three meals and two snacks per day for a week. These percentages are estimates only, and they're based primarily on my experience shopping different options in the mid-Atlantic region of the U.S. Your experience may vary according to your region and the stores you shop.

20 Percent to 30 Percent MORE: Buying at Food Co-ops

Of the options in this chapter, a well-organized food co-op is likely to have the best variety and reliability of options. They'll carry the broadest selection of prepared foods. They may even have a deli counter and a salad bar. But therein lies the reason they're more expensive than the other options. Their overhead, staffing needs, and infrastructure cost a lot to maintain.

A co-op can't offer these specialty foods in a grocery-store-like environment for the same price as a supermarket because of the limits of scale. Large supermarket chains can buy in bulk and serve a general customer. Co-ops often have only one or two locations and serve a niche customer. This is where you're most likely to encounter the noticeably higher prices that the media has told you to expect to pay for organic foods.

20 Percent MORE to 10 Percent LESS: Buying from Farmers' Markets and CSAs

In these two options, you're likely to encounter a pretty broad variety of pricing. Most of the price difference comes in the seasonality of the items.

Any fruits and vegetables are bound to be less expensive at the peak of their season when the market's loaded with them. The most expensive items from farmers' markets and CSAs will be animal products—meat, milk, eggs, and cheese—and prepared foods such as bread, cookies, and pasta.

The way to get the most for your dollar at a farmers' market is to buy fruits and vegetables at the height of the season, or slightly afterward, especially just as the next big thing is coming into season or just after the peak demand for them has passed. You may be able to strike a deal if you're willing to buy in bulk. You can also ask the farmer if he has seconds to sell. These fruits and vegetables may not look as pretty, but they're fine for soups, casseroles, and sauces.

Community Supported Agriculture programs (CSAs) can be costly in terms of the initial outlay of cash they may expect at the beginning of the season. It's not easy for working families to scrape up $400 to opt into a CSA. Others may allow a monthly pay-as-you-go option. Even though it may feel like a hefty investment, your family will be eating healthier in the long run if most of their meals are made from CSA shares, because what your farmer puts in your bag, box, or bucket will be fresh, whole foods in something very close to their natural state.

20 Percent MORE to 20 Percent LESS: Buying Directly from Farmers

Here's where the savings get more dramatic, at least when it comes to fruits and vegetables. Again, for economic reasons having to do with scale and production methods, small farmers can't offer animal products at the same prices as CAFOs. But produce is often a different story. As long as you buy in season, and especially if you buy in bulk, you can save quite a lot, simply because they have loads of it and it won't keep, and also because when you buy directly from the person who grew it, there's no middleman who needs paying, no shipping, and no warehousing costs.

The savings can get steeper if you find a farmer who delivers. Some local farmers will pool their resources and offer delivery services. The delivery charge may be as modest as $5.00 or a percentage of your total order, but many will waive the delivery fee if your order is large, or if you set up an account for a recurring order. They like regular customers and might give you a discount just for your loyalty.

Top Ten Ways to Eat Local Food for Less Than You're Paying Now for Supermarket Food

1. Eat less meat
2. Make several meals from each chicken or large piece of meat
3. Buy the seasonal avalanche and freeze it
4. Buy single-ingredient items and cook meals from scratch
5. Buy directly from real farmers
6. Plan meals around what's cheapest at the time
7. Serve a filling first course made of what's cheap, serve a smaller second course of the pricier stuff
8. Grow some of it yourself
9. Buy the farmer's seconds
10. Buy the whole cow or pig, not just the pricey cuts

10 Percent to 80 Percent LESS: Growing Some of Your Own

If you really want to offset the cost of eating fresh, local, organic produce, there's no better option than growing it yourself. In previous chapters, I've talked about the reasons why fruits and vegetables from your own backyard, balcony, or window box are the tastiest and possibly the most nutritious, and later, I'll talk about all the other intangible benefits of participating in nature's effort to provide you with food. But there's one other benefit to producing some of your family's fruits and vegetables: it's the cheapest way to get magnificently fed!

Until recent decades, the backyard vegetable patch and henhouse was the staple food source for rural low-income folk, and it still is in many parts of the world. In uncertain times, there's no better comfort than knowing that, no matter what happens in the world at large, you can come home to a larder of homegrown beans and potatoes, and eggs from your own hens.

Times have changed, and a backyard garden and home flock are not as easy to come by as they once were. Your neighbors may look askance if you replace the Jacuzzi out back with a chicken coop. Your city's zoning or homeowners' association may forbid certain agrarian activities. But there's bound to be *something* you can get away with, even if it's only a window box of homegrown lettuce.

The expensive way to garden is to go to your local big-chain home improvement store, buy market packs of prestarted plants, raised garden bed kits, brand-name fertilizers, pesticides, pots, and soil.

The cheapest way to accomplish the same thing is to compost your kitchen scraps to build great soil and save seeds from the produce you buy. They may not always germinate for you, but they're yours for no additional cost, and in any single vegetable you prepare for your family's dinner, there will be more seeds than you will know what to do with. Place them in a colander, rinse off the pulp and goo, spread them out in a pie pan, and let them dry for about a week. Then place them in a labeled bag until planting time.

Because I can't guarantee that the seeds I harvest from store-bought vegetables will grow, I also buy some of our seeds from organic and heirloom seed companies. I've had zero luck starting certain vegetables from seed, particularly tomatoes and peppers, so I buy these as seedlings from local nurseries each spring. But the more we can rely on seeds we save and organic matter we compost, the more we will save on our produce bill.

For more on this, the absolute-best option for eating locally, see Chapter 11: Growing Your Own.

Combine Sources to Get the Best Deals From Each

If you're looking to save as much money as possible—and especially, if you're like me and your goal is to eat local-organic-sustainable *for less*—your best bet is to combine the best features of all these sources.

Variety is the way to go. Try setting up weekly delivery with a local farmer for the basic staples you know your family will use: milk, eggs, bread, butter, cheese, and meats. Find a CSA or delivery service that will bring you a bag of basic produce each week, and then set yourself the challenge of using everything in the bag, even if it's something bizarre that you've never tasted before. The fact that your basics are covered means that any grocery-shopping trip is optional. This saves you money simply because, when you don't go to the store, you have zero chance of making impulse purchases.

From farmers' markets, buy whatever's in season and whatever's cheap, even if you have to buy it in bulk and freeze it.

Whenever you score a particularly wonderful item of produce from any of your sources, save the seeds! Use whatever garden space you have at home to grow as much as you can of whatever you're able to grow really well.

You can customize your use of these sources to suit your needs. Feel free to experiment until you hit upon the ideal blend of cost, convenience, taste, nutrition, and the way you prefer to spend your time and energy.

Until now, we've been talking about the price of foods from different sources. For the rest of the chapter, we'll look at techniques that will help you maximize the power of your food dollars.

Buy Whole

Whenever possible, buy single-ingredient foods in their whole, natural state. Buy cobs of corn, instead of cans of corn, and whole chickens instead of breast filets. Focus most of your food shopping on items that have a single ingredient and little or no packaging. When you buy prepared foods such as bread, cereal, or pasta, look for items that have fewer than a half-dozen ingredients, and make sure most of those added components are *food*, not laboratory creations.

Buy Non-Products

Stick mostly with foods that are not branded, copyrighted, or advertised on TV. Let your food dollars go toward *food*, not toward advertising campaigns. If you're like me and you just have to have potato chips and cookies sometimes, try to get these from local family businesses and cottage industries, or better yet, make them at home from scratch.

Shop With a Plan

Many of us blow a hefty portion of our allotted grocery budget on impulse purchases, things we didn't plan to buy, but *they just looked so good* displayed there on the store's end cap. You can head off impulse purchases by shopping with a list.

Create your grocery list by thinking in terms of meals. Shop to create breakfast, lunch, dinner, and two snacks per day, times the number of people in the household.

The one caveat to the shopping list is in the next two sections that deal with buying produce in bulk whenever it's priced low, which is usually at the height of its season. Instead of deciding in advance, "I'll buy four pounds of potatoes, a pound of spinach, and a dozen apples," leave a blank space for the specific kind of produce. Shop for four pounds of whatever starchy vegetable is seasonal (this *might* be potatoes, but it could also be yams, rutabagas, or squash), a pound of whichever leafy greens are in abundance (spinach, kale, collards, or lettuce), and a dozen of the least expensive fruit for eating out of hand (apples, plums, peaches, or pears).

The other trick to avoiding the temptation to stray from your list is to limit the number of times you shop. Try shopping for two weeks at a time, instead of once a week. The fewer times you shop, the fewer opportunities you have to come home with unplanned items.

Buy Seasonally

There are many reasons to eat food that's in season. Cost is only one. The economic law of supply and demand says that whatever the market's got too much of will be cheaper. If you know what's coming into season, you can buy up a lot of that item, plan to incorporate it into several meals a week

Five Drop-Dead-Cheap Whole Foods

Dried black beans
Dried navy beans
Dried split peas
Plain popping corn
Whole rolled oats

while the season lasts, and freeze the rest. The seasons for any given item vary according to the region in which you live. To find out what's in season at any time of year, visit www.eattheseasons.com.

Buy In Bulk Whatever's Least Expensive

Whenever you find a great deal on foods that your family uses regularly, buy a lot of them and freeze whatever you won't be able to use fresh.

The one caveat to this plan is that you want to avoid buying more than you'll be able to use. Frozen food suffers from freezer burn after a month or two. It's best to buy enough so that you're well stocked, but to keep up a healthy rotation of your freezer stock. You don't save any money at all on food that you end up throwing out because it's freezer-burned.

Most fresh produce doesn't do too well if you freeze it in its raw state. A brief boiling or sautéing will keep vegetables from getting mushy, and from losing as many nutrients. After cooking, freeze them flat in zip bags.

Best of all, you could coordinate with family, friends, and neighbors. Exchange some of your bargains for theirs. If you do this, you're practically your own miniature food co-op.

Don't Shop With Kids or On an Empty Stomach

You'll spend less if you plan your shopping trips, make a list, and avoid distractions. Shop alone if you can, because for each person shopping with you, that's one more set of impulse purchases you have to worry about. If you shop with your spouse, divvy up the list, then start on opposite sides of the store and meet in the middle.

My teenagers objected to the part about not shopping with kids. They like having a say in what we buy. Actually, there's one other extremely good reason for bringing them along: so that they can learn how to shop well. But you might want to bring them only when you're well rested, you have a little spare time, and your trip is well planned. Best of all, involve them in the planning and list-making phase as well.

Whoever ends up undertaking the shopping mission with you, make sure everyone has a good solid meal before you go. Otherwise, your hunger will persuade you to buy far more than you would on a full stomach.

Get the Basics Delivered

This is the most marvelous option for busy people, as well as for anyone on a budget. Odds are, the amount of time it saves you each week will more than offset the cost of delivery, but here's one of the best-kept secrets in the world of local foods: some small local producers will waive their delivery fee if you place a large enough order on a regular basis.

Setting up automatic delivery from local sources accomplishes a number of great things all at once. It keeps you well supplied with the good stuff and removes the temptation to impulse-purchase.

Plant a Lot of What Grows Well

After a couple of seasons of home gardening, you'll get a feel for which fruits and vegetables you can grow a lot of in the space you have available. Lettuce, potatoes, tomatoes, and zucchinis all have a reputation for burying their growers in a seasonal bonanza. Plan for an avalanche of produce!

Use What You Have

One of the side effects of paying the honest price for your food is that you're far less likely to waste it. To reduce food waste, plan to use everything you buy. Instead of running to the store for a specific ingredient, use what's on hand. If you're making a recipe that calls for asparagus and it's not in season, substitute green beans. Who knows—maybe the recipe will turn out even better.

Cook From Scratch

Buy single ingredients and combine them. You can easily make your own granola, bread, salsa, and pasta sauce. With a little practice, and a few items of special equipment, you can make your own pasta, soft cheese, and yogurt. If you have a blender or food processor, cook and purée tomatoes, dark leafy greens, and squashes, then freeze them for inclusion in soups and casseroles.

Cook in Bulk

Cook several meals at once and freeze some. Take a day when you don't have much else going on and cook for the month instead of for the day or week. Make twice as much of tonight's entrée so that it's also lunch for tomorrow. Call every rainy Sunday a baking day. Call every snow day a soup-making day. Cooking in bulk ensures that there's prepared food on hand, so even when you're on the go, you don't have to resort to buying expensive prepared meals.

Supermarket Prices vs. Local Prices: Worth a Closer Look?

In earlier chapters, I made the case that industrial food that *seems* cheap comes with hidden costs. Now, I'll share one case in which local food that appears to cost much more comes with hidden *discounts*. Last January, I had a conversation with a student—we'll call her Elaine—that went something like this:

"What do you guys pay for your local milk?"

I told her, "We pay $3.99 per half-gallon, delivered."

"Well, I just can't afford to pay that much more," she replied. "I can get it from the grocery store for $4.50 a gallon."

At first glance, that does seem like a huge difference. It would place the local option at about $3.50 per gallon *more*.

Yet there's another dynamic in this equation. The dairy that delivers our milk, meat, eggs, cheese, and bread, charges a deposit on the glass bottles in which they deliver their milk. Of each $3.99 we pay, $1.50 is a deposit on the bottle, which the dairy credits back to us when we return it the following week. That brings the price down to $2.49 per half-gallon, which means we pay 48 cents more per gallon than Elaine does.

That is, it *would* be 48 cents more, until you factor in the cost of obtaining the milk. Our dairy waives the weekly delivery fee for us, because we have a recurring order. Elaine, like all consumers who drive to the store to purchase groceries, has to pay for the gasoline it takes to schlep to the store to purchase that gallon of milk. Assuming her grocery store is less than two miles away, and assuming that she's going to the store just for the milk as we suburban moms are known to do, she spends about 34 cents in gas, effectively bringing the overall cost of a gallon of CAFO milk to at least $4.84 per gallon, compared to the dairy's $4.98 per gallon, a 14 cent difference, which is unlikely to break the bank on even the most modest food budget.

What do we get for that extra 14 cents per gallon? Milk that is free of pesticides, herbicides, hormones, and GMOs; comes from cows we know are treated right because we've *seen* them; has a better nutritional profile; tastes much richer and creamier; comes in a reusable container; supports our local community; and automatically shows up on our doorstep every Friday morning.

Cook Incredibly Filling Stuff

Focus most of your meal planning around crowd-pleasing dishes that satisfy quickly. Cook a lot of stews, soups, casseroles, and chilis. Stretch stews and chilis by serving them over rice or pasta. Cook oatmeal or grits for breakfast and top them with fruit, nuts, or homemade granola.

Cook Your Own 'Convenience Foods'

On one of your rainy baking Sundays, you could try making up a couple weeks' worth of grab-and-go lunch items, similar to the kind you used to buy at the supermarket. Burritos are quick, fun, easy to make in bulk, and can be frozen in packages of twos for quick lunches, though they will need a minute in a microwave before eating.

When you make a big batch of soup, stew, beans, or chili, freeze some of it in reusable, microwaveable single-serving containers. Wrap individual servings of quiches and casseroles in plastic and freeze them.

Eat More From Plants, Less From Animals

Only the industrial food system—with its massive government subsidies, tendency to treat animals as commodities, and focus on mass production—could possibly produce meat, dairy, and eggs more cheaply than vegetables. Anytime you see this happening, it's a result of artificial economics. When food is priced to reflect the true cost of production, fruits and vegetables will almost always cost less than animal products.

When you obtain more of your food from local sources and less from supermarkets, you'll notice right away that animal products cost more, because the food is priced realistically. Meat, milk, eggs, and cheese will claim the greatest chunk of your local food budget—that is, if they're still the centerpiece of your diet. The more you focus your food choices on plant matter instead of animal flesh, the less you'll spend.

When vegetables, fruits, and whole grains take center stage, meat becomes a sideshow instead of the main attraction. Americans are pretty atypical in the emphasis we place on meat consumption, and it's getting us into deep trouble. Your cardiologist would agree with your decision to cut back on meat and dairy. The fewer animal products you consume, the less cholesterol

Top Ten Meat Alternatives

These items are filling enough that they can take the place of a meat entrée:

1. Beans
2. Whole-grain pasta
3. Potatoes
4. Tofu
5. Eggs
6. Zucchini
7. Portobello mushrooms
8. Butternut squash
9. Peas
10. Hummus

that gets into your arteries. President Thomas Jefferson advocated a national diet in which meat should be treated as a flavoring, or as a rare treat on special occasions. If we twenty-first century Americans had followed his advice, we'd have less of an obesity crisis on our hands. On this point at least, your wallet is in sync with your waistline.

When you do cook with meat, plan to stretch it as far as you can. Buy large cuts of meat and whole chickens, then make several meals from each piece. One chicken can make a roast the first night, a casserole the second, and a soup on the third.

Cheese, which is almost 100 percent animal fat, should not be the main course in *any* dinner.

Try serving beans, peas, and whole grains alongside three or four other vegetable dishes, one of which could be a salad or a raw plate. Meat or cheese might be a flavoring in *one* of these dishes. For dessert, instead of thinking ice cream or butter-rich cookies, think mostly in terms of fruit pies, cobblers, and smoothies.

A Farmer's Advice on Price

Recently, I spoke with Mary Kathryn Barnet of Open Book Farm in Myersville, Md., about the cost of local food. I told M. K. that, in my experience, the higher upfront price of food from small, regional producers was one of the biggest concerns for consumers, and probably the single greatest deterrent for people who would like to eat local. She agreed that it was possible to feed a family on local food for the same or less as supermarket prices, but that it would take a shift in thinking to accomplish it. She told me "instead of 'what do I want to eat today?' ask yourself, 'what can I get today that's in my price range?' and then figure out how to cook it."

M. K. explained that eating local for less will often mean making alternative choices. "If you want to change the way you eat and you feel that cost is important, you probably want to cook different things," she said, "not pork chops, but the slow-cooking cuts that are less expensive. The slow-cooker is your friend."

She agrees that the best way to get a great deal on locally grown food is to purchase whatever the farmer has a lot of at any given time. When it comes to the higher upfront cost of local food, M. K. echoes what I've heard from many other farmers: that the price is higher because the food is much better quality. "It's easy to look at a dozen eggs from a supermarket and a dozen eggs from a farmer you know and think, they're just eggs. Why should I pay more? But they're not the same," she explained. "It's like comparing cotton with silk. The extra price reflects not just our labor, but the cost of feed and the processes it goes through to prepare it for sale. Ours is a better quality product."

Get Some of Your Protein From Fish

Fish is not the supercheap meat alternative it once was, and it comes with its own set of sustainability and health issues. But when you buy it carefully, it remains a high-quality, nutrient-dense, relatively low-fat source of protein. Buying carefully requires constant vigilance, as fishing conditions change frequently. As a general rule, avoid shark meat and imported seafood, even if it's farmed. U.S.-farmed scallops and trout and wild-caught salmon are a good bet, as are locally caught clams, oysters, and mussels. For up-to-date details on seafood choices, visit Monterey Bay Aquarium's Seafood Watch at www.seafoodwatch.org.

Eat Smaller But More Satisfying Portions

You may find, as you focus more of your food purchases on fresh produce and whole grains, that you're automatically eating smaller portions. When you put effort into creating a wonderful meal from fresh, whole ingredients, you tend to value it more. Instead of wolfing it down, you savor it. You eat to make it last. And, in consequence, you discover you're full before you overeat.

One way to save money on your food bill is to eat less, but that's one piece of advice nobody wants to hear. It sounds like deprivation, and we Americans just aren't into that. But without even trying to cut back on portions, if you buy the best, freshest stuff you can afford, and then you simply invest more time in preparing and eating it, you'll find that it takes smaller amounts to fill you. You'll get more pleasure and more satisfaction, even though you're eating less. That's a pretty good deal.

But If, After All This, You Still Need to Spend More to Eat the Way You Wish…

Of all the options I've presented in this chapter, there will invariably be some that won't work for you. If your family refuses to give up eating mostly meat at every meal, or if they simply can't stand to eat rutabagas three times in a week, you may not be able to hit the magic balancing point that allows you to eat local-organic-sustainable food for the same cost as supermarket fare.

No-Brainer

In his book *Fast Food Nation*, Eric Schlosser writes that, just a generation ago, 75 percent of the average family's food budget was spent on items destined to be served in home-cooked meals. Today's generation spends about 50 percent of its food budget in restaurants, primarily of the kind that markets its food as "fast."

This is why, when people who admit they eat at fast food restaurants tell me they can't afford local food, I want to smack my forehead against the nearest wall.

If you really want to eat fresh, local, sustainably grown food without increasing your food budget, this is the simplest solution of all: *you could quit going to fast food restaurants.*

You don't have to quit dining at restaurants entirely. That special meal out with the family, your paramour, or your friends brings a lot of pleasure. You could just let go of the meaningless meals-on-the-go that you end up buying simply because they're ubiquitous.

Pack something from home instead. Put that historically normal 25 percent more back into your grocery budget. Then you're eating more local food without spending any more money than you were before.

In this case, you may simply decide to raise the dollar amount you allot for food, on the notion that quality is worth paying more for. If you're on a strict budget, you might have to cut expenses elsewhere. Consider going with a cheaper cable TV company, a discount cell phone plan, or eating out at restaurants less often. If you can, make this decision as a family. Find the things that are costing you money every month but aren't bringing you much satisfaction. Rank your expenses in terms of their importance, and really consider whether each thing on that list deserves to be a higher priority than eating well.

Don't expect miracles right away. Your family might not be thrilled at the prospect of taking on more spinach and less screen time. But, as we'll discuss more in Chapter 12, humans are creatures of habit. After a while, it may feel like second nature to have great food at the heart of your home life.

Pea Soup

This soup is about the most savory, filling, healthy thing you can eat on a budget. Dried peas seldom cost more than $1.30 per pound, even organic ones. The ones you grow in your garden and leave to dry on the vine cost even less than this!

2 pounds dried split peas

1 large diced onion

1/2 pound cubed ham (optional)

Soak the peas overnight, then rinse. Place peas in a slow cooker and add enough water to cover them by a half-inch. Cook on low for 10 to 12 hours. Add water as needed to keep the peas covered to a half-inch until they dissolve. Halfway through cooking time, add onion and ham. Stir every few hours. For a fine mid-winter dinner, serve this soup with warm toasted crusty bread drizzled with olive oil.

Part 3

Learning to Eat Local: May You Live in Changing Times

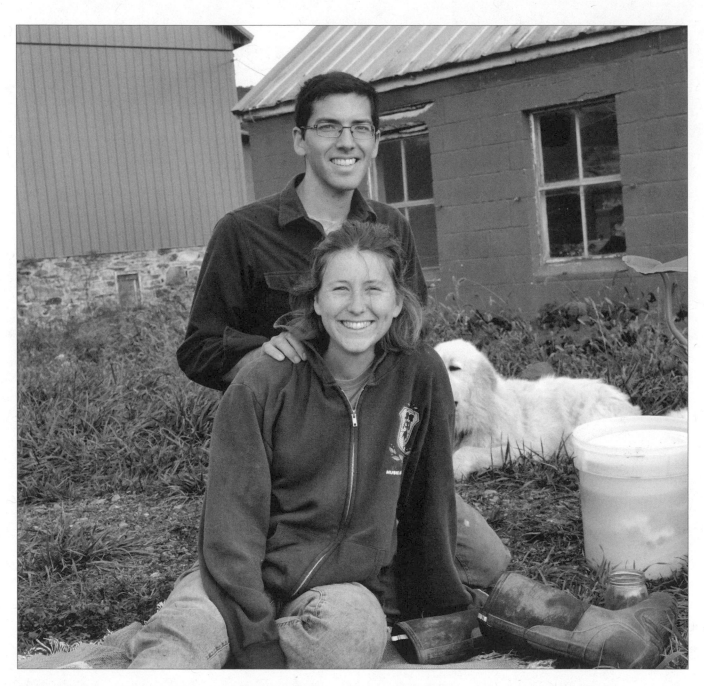

Mary Kathryn and Andrew Barnet of Open Book Farm (see page 122).

9

What to Do With It When You Get It Home

Getting Acquainted With Your Kitchen

Better a good dinner than a fine coat. —French Proverb

Golden torchlight crackled against a darkling turquoise sky. A fife-and-drum band trooped past us on frozen cobblestones, flanked by a bundled-up crowd of spectators. We stood craning our necks on wooden benches in Colonial Williamsburg two days after Christmas. Costumed interpreters set bundles of fatwood ablaze before each of the historic taverns, recited its history, and then let loose a salutary blast from their muskets.

We'd come for the annual tavern lighting—to view candles twinkling in windows, pineapples and greenery gracing doorways, and wood fires crackling in the hearths of the shops. We came to be drawn into a different era, a different rhythm of life, and of course, we came for the food.

Beside the blacksmith's shop, we found a robust outbuilding with a vast fireplace, sealed crock jars, dried herbs hanging in bunches, and the historical interpreter—a bearded man in mustard-yellow stockings—stirring a rabbit stew. While we listened to his patter about eighteenth century food, my eyes were drawn to the clay bowl full of kitchen scraps: yellowed ends of cabbage leaves, potato peels, and the stripped and boiled ribcage and leg bones of a rabbit.

At the end of his presentation, I pointed to the bowl of scraps and asked, "What would you do with those?"

"We would use up everything," he replied. He plucked a potato peel from the large bowl and placed it into an egg-sized one. "This, with a little sugar

149

and water, I would use to make yeast for bread. These," he said as he touched the cabbage leaves, "would go back into a soup. I'd take this rabbit and boil it down for stock. And the eggshells I'd put into a stocking to clarify jelly. You take the leftover jelly from the pan whenever you roast your meat. Boil it with a stocking full of eggshells. The shells suck the color and the meat flavor from it. Then you have a clear jelly you can flavor any way you like. We use everything until it's completely used up."

Each item in that bowl had a separate destiny, and every item would be used to produce more food. Even the scraps of a meal were endowed with value.

In our house, up until a year ago, leftovers such as these would have been tossed in the trash and, encased in plastic, would have made their way to the county landfill where they probably would have continued to take up space long after the demise of everyone who ate the meal that was prepared from them. In a land of plenty, we have the luxury of throwing things away.

I'd been assuming that the people who lived in colonial times cherished every morsel because food was harder to come by. Their thrift was born of necessity. But our visit to the blacksmith's cookhouse left me wondering if a society could ever adopt a value such as that, not because they had to, but simply because it's *a good one*.

Here, in the richest time and place in history, we can throw away as much of our sustenance as we like and there are still truckloads more where that came from. Obviously, abundance is better than not knowing whether there will be enough. But is it possible we've lost something intangible, unquantifiable, in the quality of our relationship with food? If we compared a meal to a love affair, the foodways of colonial folks would be a lifetime of slow, intimate tantras with a cherished partner; our ways would be a quickie in a cheap hotel room with a stranger.

What must it have been like to never take a meal for granted? Every time a colonial person sat down to eat, assuming they did more than chaw on a stump of carrot or crack open a walnut, they were eating something deliberately prepared by a person, probably by someone they knew. In the days before industrial food production, every meal represented an investment of somebody's time and energy, the product of deliberate thought and planning. Because there were no supermarkets, no interstates, and no refrigerated shipping containers, every meal had to be made of what was on hand.

Eating this way forced people into an intimacy with their food that we don't experience today. If I get up on a snowy Saturday morning and decide to do some baking, I rummage the shelves to see what we have. I don't even have an intimate knowledge of the contents of my own kitchen. And unlike these folks, who stored away several months' worth of provender, we have barely enough food in the house to make it through a week, because we can drive to the grocery store and in five minutes lay our hands on any food we want.

Freedom of choice has become absence of intimacy. In spite of all the changes we've made to our lifestyle and worldview, we are poorly acquainted with our sustenance.

In contrast, colonial people had a long-standing connection with what they ate. For most of the original inhabitants of that eighteenth century town, the relationship didn't even start at the meal, but began months earlier, with the planting of seeds and the mounding of soil. It continued through long months of rain, wind, and heat, through pinching beetles and pulling weeds. It culminated in harvesting, drying, and storing. All this they invested in during the long months before the stuff was destined to become a meal.

One other thing I noticed during our visit was the tavern menus: not the items offered to us twenty-first century tourists. These were delicious, but they were only "inspired by" genuine eighteenth century dishes. They had to be adapted to fit our modern palates or the taverns wouldn't have many customers. In late December, Chowning's Tavern served dishes with fresh zucchini and peppers, which could not have happened in an era where seasonality was imposed by the limitations of transportation.

Instead, it was the information on the *back* of the menu that really got my attention. This text described the original operating scheme for the tavern. For one thing, back in those days, you didn't get a fancy folding menu with dozens of options. Only if you were among the gentry did you come to the tavern expecting a *choice* of foods. For the everyday rabble, it was a mug of ale, a hunk of bread, and a bowl of whatever the cook could produce cheaply in bulk that evening, usually some kind of stew. Back then, nobody expected the cavalcade of choices that awaits diners even in modest eating establishments today. You ate what there was.

In the absence of much choice, they practiced a grand acceptance of a limited reality, and the result was a more intimate relationship with food than we have today.

I recognize the criticism anyone would give me if I seemed to be suggesting that we go back to eating that way: why would we *do* that? Why would we voluntarily give up fresh zucchini in December, why would we go from four dozen menu items to one, why would we waste time wringing extra utility out of an eggshell, why stick our hands in cold dirt and wait months for a harvest when we can pick up bundles of California spinach at the supermarket dirt-free anytime we want them?

Their argument makes sense on the surface. Who could deny the benefits of convenience, variety, and year-round availability? Dig a little deeper, though, and consider the true cost of these luxuries, and this viewpoint looks a little different. What it's really arguing for is our privilege *to waste*. To disconnect. To take it all for granted, as though that is our right.

Is necessity the only thing that will get us to be deliberate and intimate with our food? Or could we simply *choose it*, because in doing so we produce a deeper, more satisfying, more meaningful life?

This chapter is all about the practical aspects of developing a more intimate, conscious, and meaningful relationship with *real* food. We've talked about what it is, how to find it, and how to purchase it without taking out a second mortgage or giving up your firstborn. Now let's get down to business. We've brought this miraculous stuff into our lives for one reason: *to eat it*. To do that requires gaining a set of once-common skills that our generation has lost—yes, I'm talking about *cooking*—as well as shedding a set of expectations.

I'll share with you some of our own *aha* moments—and a few *ewww* moments—as we ended a lifetime of one-night stands with supermarket fare and began our new committed relationship with local food.

Veggie Bucket List: Try Before You Die

Snow leopard melon
Romanesco cauliflower
Parsnips
Garlic chives
Chioggia beets
Trinidad Moruga Scorpion pepper

Flat-Chested Chickens and Picasso Potatoes: Learning to Live With Food That's a Little ... Different

The local food my family is eating now is not the same stuff we used to get at the supermarket. We're aware of that eye-opening fact every day.

Most of the time, it's a happy awareness, such as the first time we cracked open pasture-raised eggs that had been inside a chicken no more than a day before we bought them. The yolks were not pale, watery yellow but a vibrant carrot-orange, and they bobbed in their clear whites like perfect little bouncy balls. My husband, Al, had read that if he cracked a pastured egg into the palm of his hand, the yolk would remain firm and round. He tried it. It really works. And the taste—exquisite!

Pastured eggs are easy to fall in love with. With other foods, it's not as easy. Grass-finished ground beef is a religious experience from the first bite, but grass-finished steak takes a little getting used to before it stirs the soul.

Pasture-raised chickens are different too, not always in an aesthetically pleasing way. They taste better, more chickeny, but the meat looks darker. The bird may have nicks in the hide or lopsided flaps of neck skin. Now and again, bits of feather might still be attached. That's how I know it was processed by hand on a small farm and not by automation in a giant factory.

At first, pastured chickens looked skinny to me, especially in the front. I had trouble getting used to eating birds that looked to my supermarket-jaded eyes like they had escaped from a weight loss clinic. Let's put it this way, if chickens wore brassieres, and the average grocery store bird was a C-cup, these lightweight ladies would probably need safety pins to hold up a training bra.

This is a classic example of the fact that what's become normal for us American eaters is, historically, not normal at all. The teeny breasts of heritage breeds are the *right* size for chickens. It's the ones in the store that are bizarre. The kind of sweater-girl roasting chicken you find at the grocery store is an industrial invention. It's likely to be a hybrid known as the Cornish Cross, the breed of chickens favored by large-scale growers and featured in Robert Kenner's film *Food, Inc.* These birds are specially raised to have gargantuan mounds of breast meat, on the notion that Dolly Parton's proportions are what consumers want (although what looks great on her isn't necessarily what we need to see on our dinner plate). They mature to market weight in only seven weeks, so quickly that their bones and organs struggle to keep up.

By giving up buxom hens in favor of the prepubescent-looking ones, we're helping to restore natural chickenness to the poultry world.

We went through a similar kind of culture shock with produce. Often, the potatoes, tomatoes, and apples we bought were comically lumpy, lopsided, or sized differently from one another. After I got used to it, I actually came to like this. I thought it gave them character. Sometimes, when we bought directly from farmers, we brought home fruits and veggies with a few small dark spots—still perfectly edible, just different. We got used to bringing home a little more dirt, a lot less packaging, and a certain amount of weirdness.

When facing the strange, we found that it helps to keep in mind the reason why everything in the supermarket looks exactly the same: because it was prepared in massive, mostly automated factories, where items must be uniform to survive the trip on conveyor belts and the long haul in shipping containers. This has nothing whatsoever to do with taste or nutrition. It has all to do with commerce.

The streamlined symmetry of mass-produced grocery store fare masks the reality of the living things that these foods once were. It's the nature of living beings not to conform to a mass-production standard. Each plant and animal is an individual. The sameness created by the factory production line erases that fact. The slightly nonstandard-shaped roasting hen we bought from a local farmer would mess up the symmetry of the production line precisely because she lived a more normal life.

I gradually came to understand the fact that the scrubbed, waxy, seemingly perfect produce that I see at the grocery store is all one shape and all one color only because that makes it more profitable to retailers, and more marketable to consumers who are still shopping with their eyes and not with their taste buds.

With a little practice, we came to love the quirkiness of genuine food—spots, lumps, wrinkles, and all.

Requisitions From the Cooking Frontier

I had a good excuse for not cooking much during the first half of my adult life. Actually, I had a string of them, mostly revolving around being too broke to afford more than ramen noodles.

First, I was in college, where being broke is part of the curriculum. Then I had twins, came to believe I'd never get a full night's sleep again, and forked over most of my paychecks in exchange for diapers and infant formula. My twins became preschoolers and I spent a fortune on Thomas the Tank Engine. I bought a house with an unusable kitchen that had been waiting for a renovation since 1960, then discovered I couldn't afford to renovate it. My twins went to school, developed the habit of chewing the erasers off their pencils, and never ate anything that wasn't slathered in peanut butter. I started teaching, thereby destroying any hope of having either money *or* time to cook. My twins became teenagers and began to leave claw marks on the refrigerator door when they came home from school. Then I married a

How to Start Cooking Actual Food

Because I'm still a pretty basic cook myself, I sought the advice of Christine Van Bloem, owner of the Kitchen Studio Cooking School, where students learn everything from the basics all the way up to advanced culinary adventures such as sushi and Thai cuisine.

Christine has helped many cooking neophytes to get comfortable in their own kitchens. I asked her what foods she recommends for people who are brand new to cooking. She said, "Start with raw foods. Learn how to cut them. The best thing you can do is to learn how to use your knife correctly."

As soon as she said this, I realized that I had no idea how I was supposed to have been holding my knife all these years. She explained that the correct way to hold a knife is to grasp both the handle and a bit of the blade—and in fact, some chef's knives have a small dent just for this purpose. "It gives you a very unsexy callus on the inside of your index finger If you do it correctly."

I asked, "Once we're holding our knives correctly, what's the next thing we need to know?"

"Cut your vegetables without killing them," she explained. "Sometimes people leave a lot of perfectly good stuff on the cutting board. Don't overdo it."

I asked her what sorts of dishes are best for people who are just beginning to cook. She recommends bruschetta, the Italian mixture of tomatoes, onions, fresh herbs, and assorted vegetables in olive oil piled onto a crisp slab of crusty bread. She likes this because it can be made without cooking. "It's a great way to just chop. It also uses up a lot of those gorgeous summer tomatoes."

Christine also has a no-cook recipe for zucchini that involves slicing it thinly, salting the slices, then tossing them in pasta with cheese. For a quick and painless way to ease into actually *cooking* some of the wonderful stuff that arrives in your CSA bag, she recommends cutting vegetables into quarter-inch or half-inch planks and grilling them. She advocates planning meals in advance: "You can't throw a meal together if there's nothing to throw. The more you plan, the better it comes off."

I asked her if she could offer any advice on how a busy person fits cooking time into a hectic lifestyle. She said, "You just have to decide you're going to make time for it, like exercising. That's how I got started. I used to go out to eat most of the time. But then I realized just how much I was missing by not cooking at home."

For anyone who's truly intimidated by the prospect of cooking, Christine advises, "People have a fear of failing in the kitchen, but there's no need to be afraid. It's just food. Assuming you live to be a hundred years old and you eat three meals a day, that's more than a hundred thousand meals in a lifetime. Even if you make a thousand bad meals, that's a tiny proportion of everything you'll eat. If you mess something up, just try it again some other time."

guy with an addiction to takeout pizza. By this time, I had forgotten what the inside of my oven looked like.

It wasn't until I made a conscious decision to make more meals at home that any of this changed. The moment that it *did* change, I came to realize that one chipped frying pan and a pizza tray wasn't going to cut it. To make home-cooked meals, I'd have to have the right tools.

At a minimum, I found I needed several large stock pots, an enormous frying pan, a couple of large casserole dishes, a roasting pan with a rack, and as many glass mixing bowls as I could cram into the cabinet. Also essential: spatulas, heat-proof stirring spoons, a slotted spoon, a ladle, a colander (that's a bowl-thingy with holes all over it for draining the water off boiled foods), and at least two really big, sharp knives.

Oh, and one other thing that I'd never owned before found its way into my life at this time: a cutting board. This item is necessary for anyone who makes meals from *food*, rather than *products*, because nearly all non-shrink-wrapped kinds of food, whatever else they may require, need to be cut up.

One of the smartest decisions I ever made was to go back to the utensil store for a second cutting board because, by owning two, I created an opportunity to work side by side with my husband or my sons, thus turning chopping time into family time.

A Time to Cook

When I talk to people about buying, growing, cooking, and eating local food, they often respond with, "well, I'd love to do that, but I just don't have the time." I understand this sentiment completely. We do live frantic, jam-packed lives. But you wouldn't have gotten this far in this book without having already made a commitment to making this change, so there must be a way to make it happen.

How did we, a typical busy suburban family of four, manage to free up enough time to cook on a regular basis? We made three major adjustments, mostly in the way we were thinking about the task of meal preparation.

First, I was lucky enough that I didn't have to take on the burden of cooking for four all by myself. In our family, we fend for ourselves for breakfasts, lunches, and snacks, with the occasional exception of a Sunday brunch, so that really left only seven dinners a week.

My husband, Al, claimed Sunday night dinner. He gets home from work so late that it isn't practical for him to cook during the rest of the week. I took Friday and Saturday, because these are the only two nights I never have an evening class to teach. My two teenage sons, after only a minimum of coaxing, fell into a routine of cooking every other weeknight. Phillip does Mondays and Wednesdays; Ben does Tuesdays and Thursdays. Anytime either one has an overload of homework, I step in and cover for them. If I have to teach that night, I make something in the afternoon that can sit quietly on the back of the stove until dinnertime. On nights when the boys have karate, whichever of them is cooking makes a casserole-type of meal that can be started, set aside for an hour, and then reheated when they get back.

One of the nicest side effects of this system was that both boys, by age sixteen, had a repertoire of about ten different meals that they could cook solo, start to finish. Not a bad skill set to be taking with them into adulthood. Someday in the not-too-distant future, a pair of nice young ladies will be thanking me for teaching this to my sons.

The second mental shift that allowed me to find the time to cook was that I decided it was something I would do as a hobby, as entertainment. By thinking of it this way, I was able to allow cooking to occupy the time I might have otherwise spent in front of the TV or on cheesy craft projects. It meant that my bead-working tools rusted, and the hand loom I never learned to use ended up covered in dust. But honestly, whipping up a wonderful meal allows me the creative outlet that I need and provides more than enough entertainment. Plus, it's nice to have a hobby that other people get some pleasure out of. My lumpy weaving projects get stashed in the backs of closets, my bracelets eventually snap and rain beads all over the floor, but my shepherd's pie gets devoured within minutes.

It's easy to enhance the pleasure of an evening spent in the kitchen. I often cook while listening to an audio book. My husband, Al, listens to movie soundtracks when he does Sunday dinners. We often cook together. We sip a glass of wine. Together, we savor the golden-orange hue of butternut squash and the heavenly aroma of garlic and rosemary simmering in olive oil. Because it's so different from all the other must-do tasks of the day—so much more immediate, visceral, and connected—it's usually the highlight of our day.

The third mental shift that has helped us turn cooking time into prime time is that we've come to view it as an excellent opportunity to interact with our kids. When I began cooking with my sons, a flood of long-forgotten memories of my own childhood resurfaced, times spent laughing in the kitchen with my mom. Trips to theme parks are quickly forgotten, but that time the marzipan dragon melted or the day the sausages kept making *that weird noise*—that's real family time.

Cooking with kids can be wonderfully fun and silly, but cooking with your mate is a whole other kind of pleasure. Don't take my word for it. Pour a couple glasses of wine, lay out all the ingredients, shoo the kids outside for a while, and find out for yourself.

First Learn to Walk, Then Learn to Fly: Start With Single Ingredients and Work Up to Recipes

We weren't entirely white belts in the cooking department when we started this experiment, but we might as well have been. The tame, overprocessed food we had been cooking for the first half of our lives bore so little resemblance to the genuine articles we were now bringing home that we felt as if we were starting over again. So we did. We started training with rookie moves and gradually worked our way up to more advanced forms.

At first, we were so deeply enamored of the beauty of the shiny orbs and giant leaves we brought home that we didn't want to do much to them for fear of messing them up. We ate many things raw. Dinner consisted of one or two cooked items, plus a large salad of cut-up peppers, cucumbers, radishes, carrots, tomatoes, whatever we had on hand. That was a good place to start, since our experiment began in early summer when we were facing an avalanche of fresh produce.

It also gave us a chance to experience the real flavors of these vegetables: ah, so *that's* what a carrot tastes like! The myth that kids hate vegetables gets perpetuated only because American kids grow up thinking vegetables are slimy dead things that come out of cans. The real truth is that when kids grow up with vegetables like *these* in their lives, they eat them with pleasure.

We graduated to yellow belt when we started cooking more of our vegetables, not as ingredients in actual recipes, but all by themselves. Kale, chard, spinach, the vibrant leafy greens were so easy. We rinsed them, removed stems, sliced, tossed them into boiling water for a few minutes, drained, and ate.

The whopping, hefty ones—squashes, eggplants, potatoes, and yams—were pretty easy, too, and we found that they made a passable meat substitute, since we were trying to reduce our consumption of animals. Summer squashes such as zucchini, crookneck, and yellow squash needed only to be sliced into thick rounds and sautéed in a little bit of butter, or cut into stout planks, dipped in oil-and-vinegar dressing, and barbecued on both sides for a minute or two. The boys went crazy for sliced eggplant dipped in a whipped egg, plopped into a dish of peppered flour, then lightly fried.

Winter squash, such as pumpkin, acorn, and butternut, can be sliced into medallions, drizzled with oil, sprinkled with salt and nutmeg, and roasted at 400 degrees. Honey, you have not lived until you have tasted roasted butternut squash!

Most root vegetables work well this way, too. Carrots, parsnips, and beets stand up to boiling, sautéing, or roasting, and they are flavorful enough all on their own to fly solo. Apples, pears, and peaches can be boiled or baked too, if you add a little honey, cinnamon, a squeeze of lemon, and maybe a couple tablespoons of flour to thicken the sauce they make with their juices. Lately, I've been topping this fruit concoction with a little granola and letting it get crisp in the oven along with whatever else is cooking.

After we had eaten these kinds of single-ingredient meals for several months, we felt ready to graduate to orange belt: simple recipes, the kind that cookbooks refer to as "level one difficulty." Among the easiest dishes at this level are casseroles, stews, and the kinds of meals that involve loading a bunch of chopped ingredients into a slow cooker set on high, covering them, and pretending they don't exist for about six hours. These are the easiest recipes to master because the ingredients just fall apart into a happy jumble. Nothing can really go wrong.

Recently, we've begun taking the next step to more complex recipes. One night I tried making a hundred-clove garlic soup (see the recipe on page 243). Rapture! I'm still trying to recover from it. Al baked an outrageous dish of egg noodles with butternut squash, garlic, white wine, and Parmesan cheese. Phillip created pure manna the day he stuffed a chicken with potatoes, portabella mushrooms, rosemary, and garlic. With us, it's all about garlic.

That's as far as we've gotten, to date. At this stage, we're beginning to catch glimpses of a future that promises adventures of the kind that can scorch, deflate, disintegrate, curdle, or light the kitchen on fire. I'll keep you posted.

Tips for Cooking Pasture-Raised Meat

Cooking with whole, fresh, sustainably raised foods calls for a few adjustments to your kitchen routine, especially when it comes to pastured meats. The website for Open Book Farm in Myersville, Md., gives this advice: "Our grass-fed animals were not raised in the same way as conventional pork, chicken, and turkey … your meat will be most tender if you allow it to thaw in the refrigerator before cooking. If you try to cook grass-fed meat that is still partially frozen, the texture will suffer."

The folks at Open Book advise making sure a cut of meat is dry before cooking so that it browns properly. They also caution consumers to cook with the correct heat for each cut of meat: "Temperature is king. There are essentially two kinds of meat: slow and fast." Slow meat, such as beef brisket and pork shoulder, turns out most flavorful and tender after long cooking with low heat. Fast meat, such as breasts and chops, needs to be cooked quickly to avoid drying out.

How Do I Cook a Nugget-less Chicken?
Preparing Whole Foods

It took some adjustment, switching from processed food-like-products to real foods. I was used to whipping foam trays of chicken breasts out of the freezer and shaking frozen potato wedges out of a plastic bag. Now I was facing a chicken that still looked like a *bird*. Whole potatoes with *things growing on them*.

I was part of this historically abnormal generation of women and men who didn't make meals from *food,* only from plastic packages. Unlike many, I was lucky enough that I learned some cooking skills from my mom when I was growing up. But then I forgot them. I've had to relearn those skills, from books, from trial and error, and from the occasional long-buried memory that suddenly swims to the surface.

If you've never faced off against a whole butternut squash or slashed your way through a mound of fresh chard, I'll walk you through some of the basics.

The first order of business is to wash the food. Meats, vegetables, and fruits alike need a good rinse, even if they're the sort of thing you peel. You want to work with clean food.

A chicken, duck, or turkey needs to be rinsed inside and out with cold water. Sorry, this is really gross, but you'll need to reach up inside the body to see if your farmer stuffed the neck or organs in there and pull them out. You can cut up the organs for gravy or soup, or feed them to the cat, but as with any meat scraps, you can't compost them. We throw ours away, and feel guilty for doing so, but we don't know what else to do with them.

Once Miss Bird is rinsed, put her on a rack inside a roasting pan, dribble a little oil over her, sprinkle the herbs and spices you like best, and roast her at 350 degrees until she is crispy and her juices run clear. If you've never done a whole bird before, you'll probably find that this is easier than you expected.

Winter squashes such as pumpkins, butternut squash, and acorn squash need to be sliced open and the seeds and pulp scooped out. Then you can slice them and bake or boil them. You'll also want to remove the skins, which is easier to do once the squashes are cooked. Summer squashes, such as zucchinis and crookneck squash, have edible skins and seeds, so all you have to do is remove the top and bottom and slice up the rest.

Unless you're baking them, potatoes need to have their eyes removed. These are the little greenish-yellow bits growing on the outside. You don't have to peel potatoes, but if you're going to mash them, you might want to do so because the peel looks weird. Boiled, baked, or fried, these things are very easy to handle and everyone loves them.

My mom taught me a trick for dicing an onion. First, slice off the top and bottom, cut a quarter-inch slit down one side, and remove the papery peel and the thickest outer layers. Then make rows of slices from the top down, cutting about three-fourths of the way through. Turn the onion ninety degrees and cut rows of intersecting slices. Then turn it sideways and slice it, this time cutting all the way through. Perfect little diced onion cubes will fall onto your cutting board.

Organically grown leafy greens such as lettuce, spinach, collards, kale, and chard need to be inspected for insect life and other hitchhikers. If you find somebody lurking on your leaves, it doesn't make the food inedible. Just remove the stowaway and rinse the leaf. You may wish to cut off the bottom portion of the stems. If you gently roll up the bundle of leaves like a loose cigar, you can then cut them crosswise with kitchen scissors or a knife, and then boil or steam them, or add them to a salad, stew, stir-fry, or quiche. Chard, that gorgeous, shiny stuff with the burgeoning red veins, cooks down far more than you might expect, so start with twice as much as you think you'll need.

Apples, pears, and similar fruits go brown after they're sliced. You can avoid this discoloration by not slicing them until mere seconds before they're eaten, or by dipping them in a mix of lemon juice, water, and sugar.

The more you work with whole foods, the more you'll learn their ways. You'll never in your life regret obtaining this knowledge. It will pay you dividends in ways that you can't imagine.

Home for Wayward Veggies

As we moved deeper into this new relationship with food, we were learning things that every housewife knew just a few decades ago: practical knowledge that served to keep the family economy on track, wisdom we've lost from our culture and now have to rediscover.

For instance, we learned that real, unprocessed food comes to us more or less in the same state it was in when it was cut from its stalk or yanked from the soil. All of the inedible bits, including some of the soil, were still attached. We had to do things to it, like wash it, chop it, and put it together with other things. And cook it, sometimes more than once.

Windowsill Radish Sprouts

If you're suffering from mid-winter gardening withdrawal, here's a quick fix. Visit your local health food store for sprouting radish seeds. Soak about a quarter cup of them in water overnight. Wash a small jelly jar and place the seeds, drained, inside. Cut a circle of plastic window screen about twice the size of the mouth of the jar and wash it thoroughly. Fix it to the top of the jar with a rubber band. Place the jar on your kitchen windowsill. Three times a day, rinse your seeds in cold water and drain them. In less than a week, you'll have fresh, spicy sprouts ready to garnish a salad. You can grow sprouts indoors year-round, even in the coldest, darkest part of winter. (Adapted from *Fresh Food from Small Spaces* by R.J. Ruppenthal.)

We also found that we have to do something with it sooner than we would have to with the produce we used to get from the grocery store. This is because the grocery store stuff was bred specially to sit for long stretches in warehouses and shipping containers, and to exude the painted-on perfection of supermodels. A lot of supermarket produce also gets sprayed with wax to prolong its fresh appearance. This wax doesn't come off. When you eat supermarket fruits and vegetables, you're also ingesting a glaze of carnauba, shellac, or resin, though some commercial grocers use petroleum-based waxes. *Yum.* Most of the local farmers I've talked to take pride in bringing their produce to the customer *unwaxed*—in virtually the same state as when it came from the field.

It sounds odd, but it's actually part of the problem with industrially produced food that it keeps practically forever. We *want* our food to be capable of breaking down, because that's how it releases its goodness to nourish other living things.

We're still learning how to use what we have while it's at its freshest. It helped to make a meal plan. Instead of grabbing every sultry, silky eggplant that winked at us seductively from the co-op shelf, we bought what we would need to make dinner, times four people, times seven nights. Food we had a plan for was less likely to go to waste.

Invariably, though, cooking like this still left a certain amount of unused food. What was I supposed to do with *one* little zucchini? Half a cup of red chard? Three carrots that wobbled when I shook them? They were still perfectly edible, and this stuff was way too expensive to waste.

To solve this problem, we learned to plan for itinerant vegetables in desperate need of immediate cooking. Through trial and error, we developed half a dozen recipes that are so flexible, we can throw almost anything into them. What follows are some of the catch-all dinners that work especially well for using up past-prime vegetables.

Shepherd's pie is the big crowd-pleaser (see the recipe on page 166). We brown a pound or two of ground meat of just about any kind (beans, tomatoes, and zucchini make a good meatless alternative), toss it in a casserole dish with several different sorts of vegetables, smear a layer of mashed potatoes on top, and bake for about half an hour at 400 degrees. Peas, carrots, and onions are the standard trio for this dish, but I have yet to find a veggie that doesn't work in shepherd's pie. Chard, zucchini, corn, and even weirdos such as parsnips are welcome. One of my favorite things about shepherd's pie is that it lends itself nicely to the old-fashioned spices I seldom use in any other dish: coriander, savory, and marjoram. It's charming. It's filling. It's simple. No matter how much I make of this stuff, there are never any leftovers.

Chicken stew is another great place to make use of mismatched veggies. We usually plan to make this on the day after we've roasted a chicken, as a way to use up the leftover meat. We boil the leftover chicken frame in a half gallon of water for a few hours. Then we remove the frame and strain the broth through a colander to remove any bones. We cut the remaining meat off the frame and return the meat to the broth. We bring the broth to a boil, toss in a nice whole-grain pasta, and let the pasta cook until it's tender, then we add a little milk, butter, and flour. Finally, in go whatever veggies we have on hand. The only veg that doesn't work well here seems to be potatoes, but that could just be me. A variation on this theme is to throw the whole thing into a casserole dish, grate Parmesan cheese over it, and bake it like a casserole.

Another great place to park the odd veg is in a stir-fry. Into a large pan with olive oil, we toss chopped vegetables according to which ones take the longest to cook. We start with the burly ones such as carrots and onions, segue to the broccolis and zucchinis, and finish with tomatoes, mushrooms, and any kind of sprout. We add beef, chicken, sausage, or tofu, and serve the whole thing over rice or noodles.

My personal favorite catch-all dish is quiche, partly because it's nearly impossible to mess up. It takes about fifteen minutes to make the crust (I confess I usually use store-bought pie crusts for quiches because my home-made crusts taste like wallpaper paste). I beat about seven eggs per quiche with a half cup of milk, add a little herb or pepper, and toss in some cubed cheese and a cup of whatever veg is most in need of TLC. Then I bake it at 350 degrees until it goes a little bit golden-brown on top.

When we plan on two or three of these kinds of meals each week, we're able to find a home for that lonesome quarter of an onion drying out in the back of the fridge, as well as most of its fellow outcasts. It took some trial and error to get there, and an awful lot of past-prime produce went into our compost heap in the meantime. We found we had to make a paradigm shift from cooking specific recipes to building meals out of whatever was threatening to go wrinkly first.

Regarding geriatric veggies, a word to the wise about your teenage chefs, who will cook and will usually do so happily and creatively. But left to their

The Life Span of Local Vegetables

When you're eating genuine fresh, local produce, you'll need to organize your weekly eating plan around what needs to be consumed soon. Here's how long you can expect fresh foods to last, assuming refrigeration or cool storage:

Eat Within 1 to 2 Days: Spinach, kale, broccoli, salad greens, fresh corn, berries, sprouts, bok choi, asparagus

Eat Within 3 to 5 Days: Carrots, eggplant, cauliflower, tomatoes, avocados, green beans, peaches, pineapples, bananas, peppers, peas, cucumbers, radishes, herbs

Eat Within 1 to 2 Weeks: Garlic, leeks, parsnips, beets, rutabagas, summer squash

Eat Within 1 to 2 Months: Winter squash, potatoes, cabbage, onions, apples, pears

Eat Within 4 to 6 Months: Honey, nuts, seeds

own devices, they will choose to cook the best stuff on hand, not the items that ought to be used within the next day or two. I learned the hard way that when I share cooking duty with the rest of the family, I'm the one who ends up with the task of finding a use for the flaccid celery and elderly green beans. I've come to view it as a challenge, as one more way of closing the environmental loops we've left dangling for so long, and maybe even, in a weird way, a form of charitable service for vegetables less fortunate.

An Infestation of Dirty Dishes

Now for the most distressing part: When you cook every day, you make an ungodly number of dirty dishes. It's incredible. I can literally empty the sink down to the last fork the night before and have the whole thing so filled-up again by the next day that I can't even get a glass of water from the tap.

The reason for this avalanche of greasy cookware is that now *we're* doing all the processing that who-knows-how-many factories used to do for us. Unless we're prepared to eat carrot sticks and apple wedges every night, something's got to be done to the stuff, and that dirties a lot of cookware.

I wish that I had some brilliant bit of advice for you about this, but I don't. I'm still struggling. My teenagers will do dishes, but usually only when asked, and they have this way of conveniently not seeing the greasiest pans. My husband sometimes comes in the door at 7:00 p.m. and goes straight to the sink to get a load into the dishwasher before dinner. I don't think that's particularly fair—he has a long commute—but a sink full of greasy dishes drives him crazy.

It's a problem, and not just because, as a chore, it ranks right up there with cleaning the litter box. It uses up a lot of water and electricity, and it dumps detergent into the septic system. Disposable kitchenware isn't the answer. We don't want to add more to the waste stream. Maybe someday, a genius will invent compostable cookware. Until then, if you have any solutions for the dirty dish dilemma, please e-mail me and let me know!

Oh, the Feasts You'll Make!

Once we settled into the notion of cooking for ourselves, we made an astonishing discovery: *cooking makes us happy!* We learned to approach it not as a daily, get-it-done chore, but as a chance to play, with the added bonus that at the end of playtime you get to eat something amazing.

Fixing and eating home-cooked food delivers many kinds of bliss, on many levels. The pleasures of eating this way start long before the meal and linger long afterward. First of all, it feels nice to cook for someone you love. It's a gift to invest time and creative energy in making great food for friends and family. Then there's the sensual dimension: the color, aroma, and taste of the food, the feel of it between the fingers. There's the time spent together consuming it. And then there's more. When you eat this great stuff, you feel better.

Al sometimes fixes an aromatic vegetarian chili with sautéed cumin seeds, zucchini, tomatoes, curry paste, and a whole carnival of vegetables. While it's cooking, the whole house smells like an Indian restaurant. The flavors of this thing are so elegant; the textures are so complex. No french fry could compare with the song this stuff plays on my tongue. But the best part comes the next day, and lasts for a few days afterward. My mind is clearer. I have more abundant, cleaner-burning energy. If you struck me with a mallet, I'd ring like a chime.

Few investments can return the kind of rapture, connection, and satisfaction that come from homemade feasts made with real food. When I eat this way, when I feed my loved ones like this, I feel a deep sense of happiness, well-being, belonging in the world, and optimism about the future.

Whatchagot Shepherd's Pie

4-6 large peeled potatoes

1/4 cup milk or soymilk

1/4 cup olive oil

2 pounds pastured ground turkey or beef

1 large onion

2 cups vegetables of your choice, in any combination, whatever needs to be used up

4 cloves garlic

1 cup gravy (optional)

1 teaspoon coriander seeds

1 teaspoon marjoram

1 teaspoon savory

1 teaspoon paprika

Boil and mash the potatoes, add milk as needed to soften the mash. In a very large skillet, fry ground meat in olive oil along with the garlic and spices. Add gravy and stir. Place the contents of the frying pan into a large casserole dish and smooth it down.

Slice the vegetables thin and lay them atop the meat. Layer the mashed potatoes on top. Sprinkle the potatoes with paprika. Bake for about 45 minutes at 350 degrees, until the potatoes begin to turn golden.

10

Four Seasons of Eating Locally

Or, Why It's Weird to Eat a Tomato in January

Live each season as it passes. Breathe the air, drink the drink, taste the fruit, and resign yourself to the influences of each. —*Henry David Thoreau*

B ut how do you feed yourself in the winter?" This is the question many people ask when they find out about our local food experiment. Even hard-core supermarket shoppers have enough agrarian awareness to notice that their neighbors' vegetable gardens go brown and wrinkly when cold weather sets in. How can we eat locally grown food when the soil is frozen so hard it rings like a stone when you hit it, and the only thing that's growing is the monthly heating bill?

We discovered part of the answer to this question during our Christmas-time visit to Colonial Williamsburg a couple of years ago. Following cobblestone streets, we strolled past holly-swagged doorways graced with pineapples and dried orange slices. I couldn't help noticing how many tidy kitchen gardens grew behind white picket fences: carefully edged, crisscrossed with oyster shell pathways, mulched for winter in straw or pine needles, but incredibly, still growing in late December.

At that time, my own garden back home consisted of four purpling broccoli plants, three withered cabbages struggling to wrap themselves into ping pong ball–sized heads, three spindly celery stalks, and a box of carrots the size of golf tees that were only beginning to show the tiniest ghost of orange. Here in Williamsburg, lettuce and spinach leaves still flourished glossy summer green, fat globes of purple and white rutabagas muffin-topped their way out of the soil, and the stout orange roots of carrots glowed under feathery green foliage. How were they doing this?

It probably helped that they were a five-hour drive south of where my winter garden was struggling for survival. It certainly also made a difference that their gardens were tended by staff and volunteers who knew what they were doing, instead of one overextended college instructor. But as I looked closer, I saw the most marvelous techniques at work. Over the newest seedlings, they had placed thick glass bells with knobs on top. These gathered the weak winter sunlight and concentrated the moisture. In places, these historical botanists had woven short fences out of twigs, perhaps to protect the tender plants against winter wind. Everywhere, rows of plants grew from within thick, comfy blankets of mulch. The whole effect was one of loving, deliberate attention.

If the "how do you feed yourself in winter" question had been posed to the original colonial-era folks, if they had been asked how they managed without fresh food for months at a time, their answer would have been they didn't. They had less of it, to be sure, in January than in July, but they were solicitous enough to the needs of their vegetables to know how to coax at least a few of them into growing year-round. Just as they had a plan for deriving nourishment from spring's sprouting, summer's lushness, and fall's bounty, they were practiced hands at feeding themselves through the lean, cold months of winter. An intimate knowledge of the cycles of nature meant you could tap into at least some sources of sustenance, regardless of the time of year.

If you're moving to a way of eating that's in harmony with the way nature produces food, you quickly come to realize that food is seasonal. Food has seasons because nature has seasons, and real food comes from nature. Processed food doesn't have seasons because factories aren't part of nature. A hundred years ago, and in all previous eras, no one needed to have this explained to them, because they lived it, in the same way that they lived the sun going down in the evening and rising again in the morning. But today, we've allowed the year-round availability of foods in supermarkets to influence our taste buds. We've lost touch with the simple fact that food tastes best when it's in season.

My grandma knew that asparagus came around in May, strawberries in June, and apples in September. She understood that eggs tasted less vibrant in winter because the hens were missing out on all the bugs and worms that make their eggs so flavorful. To Grandma's generation, and all those before hers, eating seasonally was *normal*. There was simply no other practical way to do it.

We lost our awareness of seasonal harvests when we began to eat foods that could survive a thousand-mile trek across the country and a year-long wait in a warehouse. We cut short our intimate connection to the seasons when we began importing Brussels sprouts from Mexico in winter and grapes from Chile in the spring. Asparagus spears with tomato slices, although a heavenly combo, is a seasonal aberration, as unnatural as parrots romping with polar bears.

You may be thinking, what's wrong with getting my lettuce from California during the parts of the year when my own lettuce patch is frozen under a slick coating of ice? It's certainly not a sin, but it's not without cost that your California lettuce finds its way to you. Transporting your lunch around the country takes fuel. Petroleum burned to transport something that can be grown locally is fuel that is used needlessly.

It also takes packaging. The locally grown lettuce that sits in a bushel basket at your local farmers' market for just a couple of hours before you buy it requires no package. The California lettuce needs to be protected from dirt and moisture on its long travels, so it comes to you sheathed in a plastic sleeve that will long outlive the head of lettuce it protects, and also the people who eat the lettuce, as well as their children and grandchildren.

Not only this, but most produce is pretty fragile. It doesn't survive all that packing, shipping, and warehousing without taking a hit in the quality department. Red Delicious apples—in my opinion, the world's most tasteless fruit—were bred to sit in a warehouse for long periods of time. Despite their yummy-sounding name, their leathery skin and mealy flesh taste about as flavorful as the cardboard cartons they're shipped in.

Some of the reasons for eating *seasonally* are subtle. Take, for instance, the idea that eating in accordance with the rhythms of the seasons leads you into a deeper relationship with the natural world. Respecting the seasons teaches humility. Sure, we can grow a tomato in a greenhouse in January, but we can't equal the radiant energy of a ruby-red tomato picked off the vine in the baking hot sun of July. Knowing our limitations reminds us that even though we do know it *some*, we don't know it *all*. We can live to pillage nature, to compete with it, to attempt to dominate it, or we can live within its mystery and complexity—open to the possibility that there's quite a bit more to the natural world than we have yet discovered.

Eating seasonally is worth doing for reasons of ecology and economic fair play, but if you're thinking that you'll be giving up something when you switch to a seasonal diet, you're in for a surprise. Eating in harmony with the seasons doesn't detract from your enjoyment of food; *it adds to it*. It contributes an exquisite layer of pleasure to your life.

How does it do this? By adding anticipation to your gastronomic experience. You can't just have a particular kind of food any old time you crave it. You have to wait until its time has come. It's Christmas morning. It's the "ready" light on the waffle maker.

Not only that, you're now privy to a secret that only seasonal eaters know: food is at its most rapturous, its most flavorful, when it's at the peak of its season. Fresh fruit and vegetables in season are so delicious that their arrival is an occasion in and of itself. When you eat this way, your calendar fills up with many more exciting events to look forward to: the first blueberries of the year, the first spring onions, and the earliest baby lettuce. Something's always coming into season, something's always on its way, a whole year of pleasures on the horizon.

Just so you're clear about where I stand on the issue, I'm not categorically opposed to *all* produce shipped in from outside my region. My family occasionally eats oranges and bananas—we've never seen *these* growing in Maryland—and we do supplement our winter food supply with a small amount of produce from points south. Given the current reality we live in, it would be difficult for those of us who live in colder climates to take an all-or-nothing stance when it comes to local eating. Our goal in winter is the same as in all other seasons: to choose local foods as often as we can.

What Grows When: A Primer for the Veg-Illiterate

To us humans, a "vegetable" is the edible part of a member of the plant kingdom, those organisms that have a cellular structure, produce energy from photosynthesis—that's what makes the plants green—and reproduce sexually. Most, but not all, of the plants we eat are angiosperms, meaning that they reproduce by flowering.

Most of the plants you find growing on farms or in home vegetable gardens are domesticated species of angiosperms, with a long history of symbiosis with humans. To say that a plant is domesticated means that humans have selectively bred it, over many generations, to have the traits we like. Corn, wheat, tomatoes, and many other staples of the modern human diet are so far removed from their wild ancestors that they bear about as much resemblance to them as a tabby cat does to a tiger. Over time, we've bred our domestic vegetables to serve us, and they've been rewarded for their cooperation by flourishing in our care.

The "edible" part of the definition is important because, in many of the domesticated plants we eat, some parts are delicious and some will kill you. In other words, before you chow down, it's good to know which parts are the edible ones.

What's In Season When

These fruits, vegetables, herbs, and nuts are available locally in season in most of the continental United States.

Winter	Spring	Summer	Fall
beet	asparagus	basil	apple
broccoli	artichoke	beans	artichoke
carrot	blackberry	cantaloupe	broccoli
chard	blueberry	corn	cabbage
kale	carrot	cucumber	carrot
mushroom	chard	eggplant	cauliflower
parsnip	cherry	fennel	celery
potato	chive	green bean	chard
rutabaga	dill	melon	cranberry
turnip	fennel	onion	fig
winter squash	leek	oregano	garlic
	lettuce	peach	grape
	mint	pepper	hazelnut
	new potato	plum	kale
	radish	raspberry	okra
	rhubarb	summer squash	parsnip
	spinach	tomato	pear
		watermelon	peanut
		zucchini	potato
			shallot
			winter squash

To do that, you have to know your way around a plant. During its life span, any given plant is made up of these parts: sprouts, roots, stalks, leaves, flowers, fruits, and seeds. Which of these bits your veggie has is a function of what stage of growth it's in. All our vegetables start life as seeds and sprout into seedlings, typically producing one or more thin roots below ground and two chubby baby leaves above ground, before growing their "grown-up" leaves and roots. The seedlings grow and develop larger stalks and more leaves, along with thicker roots under the soil. Eventually, they flower. If their flowers are pollinated, they make fruits, which, when ripe, contain the next generation of seeds.

Seeds, sprouts, roots, stalks, leaves, flowers, fruits—we may eat any of these, depending on the kind of vegetable. We eat the seeds of corn, peas, beans, cereal grasses, and sunflowers. We enjoy the sprouts of radishes, alfalfa, broccoli, asparagus, and beans. We eat celery and rhubarb stalks. We grow spinach, chard, lettuce, kale, and collards for their leaves. We like the flowers of broccoli, cauliflower, and artichoke. With some veggies, it's the part under the ground that we crave. That's the case with potatoes, carrots, rutabaga, radishes, peanuts, and turnips. With others, the only parts we can safely eat are the fruits—for instance, the fruits of eggplant, tomato, and pepper. The rest of the plant is poisonous. If you've ever heard of deadly nightshade, you might be amazed to find that it's the edible fruits of these and other members of *solanaceae,* the nightshade family, that you're dining on.

If you want to stay alive, it's a good idea to know what part is edible on each veggie you wish to consume. With some plants, such as beets, the whole thing can be eaten: roots, stalks, and leaves. With others, certain parts of the plant are toxic, such as the leaves, stems, and roots of tomato, eggplant, and pepper, or the leaves and roots of rhubarb.

With few exceptions, each of these edible plant parts has its season. Seeds sprout in early spring, flowers emerge in late spring, fruits emerge in early summer, and then the plants spend most of the summer growing roots, fruits, and leaves. The bigger the fruit or root, the longer it takes to finish growing. The consequence of this natural cycle is that different foods have their seasons. The time of year to enjoy sprouts, shoots, and baby salad greens is spring. The season for big, broad leaves and small fruits such as strawberries and blueberries is early summer. Peppers, tomatoes, eggplants, and soft-skinned summer squashes such as zucchinis come along in high summer, along with most of the stone fruits such as peaches and plums.

Late summer and early fall bring apples and potatoes. Late fall is the time for big winter squash, such as pumpkins, and thick root crops, such as turnips.

The timing and length of seasons varies according to the region in which you live. The further north, the later, and probably shorter, the seasons will be for many of your favorite fruits and vegetables.

With that thought in mind, let's tour each of the seasons with an eye to what to look forward to eating.

Spring

In the mid-Atlantic states, where I live, spring is about as punctual as a weekend plumber. It gets there when it gets there. No amount of pointing out the date on the calendar makes any difference. One year, the forsythias are bursting by the last week in February, then the next, it's early April and you've got an inch of snow on the daffodils. Around the Washington, D.C., area, we love to smirk at the fact that the Cherry Blossom Festival rarely seems to coincide with the arrival of the blossoms.

If the weather's good, backyard gardens in the middle latitudes of the United States might see a smidge of action by mid March. The garlic I snuck out of the fridge and planted there last fall is already up, the onion bulbs and seed potatoes go into the ground, and we might throw around a few handfuls of carrot and radish seeds. In 2014, the last day of March bore a close enough resemblance to spring that I risked planting some of the cold-weather things I'd started indoors: spinach, kale, peas, lettuce, dill, chard, and rhubarb. Some of it survived.

In the mid-Atlantic, April brings a few fresh salad greens, the earliest spring onions, asparagus, rhubarb, and the first tenuous openings of local farmers' markets. But nothing really gets rolling until May.

Early spring is an especially good time for remembering that there's a natural world out there. Even the most tuned-out urbanites notice the first flashes of emerald green, and the sparkle of yellow and violet from the first bulbs to emerge. People who think they possess zero plant lore come to discover they have at least a little. Something about early spring brings back a surge of long-forgotten memories about wild food gathering.

As I fell deeper and deeper in love with local foods and farming, I redis-covered my own foraging memories. When I was growing up, my great Aunt Leona, who would otherwise never go near anything that could be called

You Know It's Spring When...

... these early spring vegetables start appearing in your local farmers' market or CSA bag:

Asparagus
Baby lettuce
Pea shoots
Rhubarb
Spring onions

nature, would gather us up on just the right spring day, order us all into galoshes, hand out plastic bags, and herd us out into the woods to gather poke. This is the stuff that, when it gets old enough to develop the wine-colored stem and berries, is poisonous, but if you know how to spot it when it's young enough, it tastes like spinach from the gods. Even when we picked it young, I remember Aunt Leona had to boil it for a long time, in several changes of water, to make it safe to eat. It's known by the old-time folk for having certain beneficial effects which I'll leave to your imagination, except to say that it gives new meaning to the term "spring cleaning."

I grew up in a time and place where all the young folk had free rein to traipse around in the woods. The neighborhood kids I hung out with often amused themselves by doing a little wild foraging. I ate my fair share of wild strawberries in spring and mulberries—green bugs and all—in summer. I sucked the one teeny drop of honeyed nectar from the end of a honeysuckle blossom, and then wore the small, sticky green cone at the flower's base on the end of my nose. It was what we did for fun back then, before the Internet.

I dated a guy in high school who had trained himself on wild food lore by talking to old-timers and reading the *Foxfire* books, the collection of Appalachian wisdom compiled by Eliot Wiggington and his students. He showed me how to find joe-pye weed, partridge peas, sassafras, onion grass, and a golden-lobed fungus he called a chicken mushroom, which I refused to go near. I was a little squeamish about tasting the wild plant foods he'd gathered, so he would sneak some of them into whatever I was eating and then tell me later that I had eaten it. He once gave me a cup of what he had told me was Red Zinger tea, but which later turned out to be stag horn sumac. He also showed me, one late February afternoon, a patch of spring beauties: tiny blue five-petaled flowers, among the earliest plants to start growing with the return of the sun. He dug some up and held out the pearly bulbs that grew just below the surface. They looked and tasted just like miniature potatoes. To this day, I mark the official start of spring by the day I notice the spring beauties spangling the grass.

According to the *Foxfire* books, the folks who fed themselves by their own labors saw the first days of spring as signs of hope. They were furtive seed-savers, and the previous autumn, had carefully dried and stored the best seeds from the summer's crop. In spring, these would be carefully deployed into well-manured soils, each according to its time. Then they waited on sunshine and warm rain showers.

Summer

The absolute best time to become a local eater is summertime. At this time of year, you won't need to research to find farmers' markets. Just toss a rock in the general direction of town on a summer Saturday morning and you'll hit a few. Neighbors with an overload of backyard produce will be setting it out on folding card tables at the ends of their driveways, maybe with cash boxes for honor system donations or signs that say "Free—take some—*please!*"

If you love fresh fruit, from June to September you'll be livin' large. In the mid-Atlantic region, early June brings strawberries, in late June come blueberries and cherries, and then in July, blackberries. Peaches and plums come along in July and August, and grapes in September. The first apples may come as early as June, but most will arrive in the fall.

A similar story unfolds with vegetables. Lettuce is best in May, and spinach and kale arrive around this time, too. You'll bite into your first tomato in late June, along with the earliest peppers. July brings the first zucchinis, yellow squash, cucumbers, beans, and eggplants. All the warmest weather vegetables start as a trickle and end the warm season as an avalanche, which brings us to the next season.

Harvest

Feng shui, the ancient Asian belief that the natural world is influenced by a force known as chi, recognizes *five* seasons, not four, one to correspond with each of the five elements. Between summer and autumn comes harvest. Harvest begins with the first frost, when the garden plants get their first whiff of their own mortality, launch into overdrive, and bury their gardeners in an avalanche of late-season produce. They do this just when many of the other crops that take a full season to mature—the winter squashes, the apples, and the potatoes—suddenly come into readiness. What we have here is a full-on end-of-season produce attack, a rampaging Foodzilla. This is the key time to buy in bulk. You'll be able to get the year's best foods in a colorful avalanche of goodness. This is when, if at all possible, you want to set aside time to can, freeze, dry, and store your bounty.

I've never actually tried to can anything, so I can't speak to you about it from experience. I've been told that there are two kinds of canning: the

Wines That Pair Well With Summer Produce

Apricots: Sauterne

Corn, Lima beans, melons: Chardonnay

Green beans, zucchini, kale, collards: Sauvignon Blanc

Plums: Oloroso sherry

Tomatoes: Chianti, Cabernet, Sangiovese

safe kind that involves tomatoes and vinegars and such a high acid content that nothing can grow inside the jar, and the scary kind that involves special pressurized equipment and more know-how than I've got.

If canning seems like an iffy prospect, or like way too much work, you can get similar results from freezing. Most of your produce will need to be blanched (boiled briefly) or sautéed in order to survive the freezing process without becoming brown mush. Slice larger veggies into slabs, cook lightly, cool them on a rack, and then stick the rack in the freezer. When the slabs are frozen, you can pack them into reclosable freezer bags. You can buy plastic bags that attach to a little battery-operated gizmo that sucks all the air out of the package and protects your food from freezer burn, or you can accomplish results almost as good the low-tech way—by inserting a plastic straw into a corner of the bag and sucking out the air by mouth before you seal the bag all the way.

Drying is also a reasonable way to preserve your harvest. I dry mint, basil, rosemary, parsley, and cilantro in little bundles over my kitchen sink throughout the growing season. I hang them top-down, to keep the oils in the leaves, until they're dry and brittle. Then I remove the stalks, crumble them, and seal them in jelly jars I've washed to reuse. Apples, pears, and pumpkins will dry nicely if you slice them thin and put them on a tray in a very low-heated oven, about 200 degrees, but that takes gas or electricity. Country folk used to string such things on cotton twine and hang them up on a rafter somewhere to air dry. They used to do a similar thing with green beans, passing a needle and thread through their sides to make a long, hanging garland. If you acquire your garlic and onions with their dried green tops still on, you can braid them into long, gorgeous bundles to hang in your kitchen. Who needs cheesy store-bought kitchen décor when you can array your home with the season's bounty?

Autumn

Autumn is probably the best time to visit local farms. The harvest is in, so farmers aren't putting in the sunrise-to-sunset hours that they were just a few months earlier. They can relax and chat with visitors. By this time of year, fruits and vegetables have absorbed a full season's worth of sunshine and nutrients, and they're sitting back, gorged and sated. If you could put a word on the feeling that settles over farms at this time of year, it would be *accomplishment*.

Fall Veggies That Keep a While

Cabbage
Parsnips
Potatoes
Rutabagas
Winter squash

In late fall, farmers have no shortage of the kinds of hearty fare that stores well over winter: potatoes, yams, winter squashes, onions, and cabbages. If you come across a bounty of these foods, by all means, grab them up by the bagful. They will sit happily in a basket or box in your basement or garage, wrapped in newspaper, or on a cool porch, buried in straw against freezing. Cover them well and keep them away from water, critters, and extreme cold, and they're likely to stay edible the whole winter.

Avid home gardeners can often be found putting one last round of autumn vegetables into the ground in early September. Spinach does well this time of year because it likes to start in warm soil, but it can keep struggling along well after the first frosts. Broccoli, celery, cabbage, and carrots can also reward your efforts long into November and beyond, depending on where you live.

Winter

Through this chapter, you've probably been thinking, sure, it's not that hard to eat seasonally during the growing season, but what about the dead of winter? How will I eat seasonally when there's nothing green outside? I can't just swear off food from December to March.

You're right that it's harder to eat locally during the winter months. It can be more expensive, too. But if you're willing to do a little investigating and a little experimenting, that—plus the wondrous bounty you canned, froze, and dried a few months before—will get you by.

The first winter after our decision to eat locally, we assumed that we'd have to break our own rules during the winter. And in perfect honesty, we did buy mostly California-grown produce before we figured out how to tap local sources. It took more than half the winter to find a farmers' market that stayed open year-round. I lost a crop of indoor carrots to carrot flies and a crop of indoor rosemary to the cat before I began to get the hang of indoor winter gardening. But gradually, our sources of fresh local winter sustenance grew.

Most of our sustenance that winter came from our local food co-op, which tries to obtain as much of their produce as possible from local sources but does import a fair amount of their winter fare from organic California growers. We won't beat ourselves up about it. After all, it was our first winter trying to do this.

What Grows in Alaska and Hawaii

Because of the distinctive climates in Alaska and Hawaii, their local offerings differ greatly from the rest of the United States. In Alaska, produce is grown in greenhouses during much of the year. Hawaii grows many of the same fruits and vegetables available elsewhere, in addition to some of its own unique offerings.

Alaska	Hawaii
barley	coffee
blueberries	kiwi
broccoli	lychee
Brussels sprouts	macadamia
cabbage	pineapple
carrots	rice
cauliflower	sugarcane
quinoa	sweet potato

Five Massively Healthy Winter Foods

Alfalfa sprouts
Black bean soup
Pea soup
Sauerkraut
Winter squash

If we had been smarter about stocking up while the good times were rolling—that is, during harvest time—we'd have had a fuller freezer, a fuller wallet, and more options. But we did find a few ways to amuse ourselves while we waited for the natural world to show signs of life. We played in the kitchen. We spent the winter months experimenting with recipes. Twice, I grew fresh radish sprouts in a jelly jar. Plus, we got about two cups of salad greens per month from the window box I parked on the kitchen windowsill. We'll be wiser and better prepared next winter.

So how does the local eater's year differ from that of the person who shops at the local supermarket day in and day out? Both the local farm patron and the supermarket shopper are subject to the same mercurial climate and the same shifts in light, weather, soil, and season. But only the seasonal eater experiences these transformations intimately. The supermarket shopper lopes steadily through all four seasons, unaware. In the grocery store, one season is pretty much like the next, but for the local eater, the landscape transforms nearly every week. Each season has its trials and joys, anticipations and rewards, and booms and busts. The seasonal eater knows there's always something to be thankful for, and always something to look forward to.

Parsnip Pudding Pie

I know they're funny looking, but they're quite possibly the sweetest-tasting vegetables on Earth. In centuries past, both here and in Europe, they were *the* fall vegetable of choice. When I taste mashed parsnips with butter, I think of eggnog and custard tarts. I always wanted to see what these weird old-fashioned vegetables would do if I put them in a dessert, so I did a little experimenting. Try this if you're feeling brave.

1 deep dish pie crust

4 large peeled boiled mashed parsnips

3 eggs

1/2 cup cream

1/2 cup honey

1 teaspoon vanilla extract

1/2 teaspoon nutmeg

pinch of ginger

Run the mashed parsnips, about half of the cream, and vanilla extract through a blender or food processor until very smooth. Beat the eggs. Add the parsnip mixture, the rest of the cream, honey, nutmeg, and ginger and stir thoroughly. Empty the mix into the pie crust. Bake at 325 degrees for 30 minutes or until the pie quits being jiggly in the center. If your kids ask what's in it, explain that you'll only tell them after they've tasted a bite.

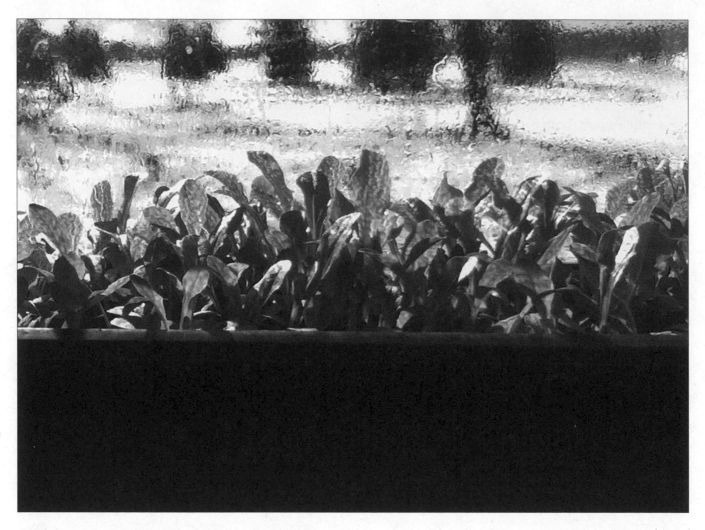

Fresh lettuce growing on the author's windowsill.

11

Growing Your Own

You Can't Get More Local Than This

Though an old man, I am but a young gardener. —*Thomas Jefferson*

Granddaddy came from North Carolina farming folk. I visited his family's farm a few times when I was a kid. Several generations of the family still live on that land, grandmas and nephews and cousins, all a ten-minute walk from each other.

When I was tiny, I loved running along the grassy pathways in Granddaddy's rose garden, with a carnival of brightly colored blooms towering above me. I'm sure time has warped the image, but in my memory, those rose bushes are eight feet tall.

Last summer, when I successfully grew my own tomatoes for the first time, I remembered Granddaddy picking tomatoes out of his garden, grabbing a salt shaker, and biting into one of those juicy red globes as if it were an apple. I can't remember things that happened in my twenties and thirties as well as I can recall the ecstasy on his face as he savored a tomato that had been growing on the vine minutes before. And now I could enjoy my own tomatoes the same way.

I told my mom about my tomatoes.

"I'm so glad you're into gardening, Jul. Your grandfather would be so proud."

Wow. Nothing I had ever managed to do had gotten me much of a blip on the family-pride radar. Not graduating college. Not writing books. Not getting married or having kids or any of the usual things that seem to make a mom proud. But in growing tomatoes, I finally became a credit to my heritage.

My generation is the first to depart from a food-growing tradition. Most

Never Have So Few Fed So Many

The United States Census estimated the total population of the United States at 313,873,685 for the year 2012. According to the United States Bureau of Labor Statistics, the number of people employed in farm-related industries in the country that same year was 427,670, or fewer than 2 percent.

American families in previous eras knew how to raise a few things at home, if only a humble potato patch out back or half a dozen laying hens under the porch. During the Civil War, the Great Depression, World War II, and indeed throughout most of this country's history, Americans have responded to tough times by growing more of their own sustenance, supplementing store-bought groceries with simple food that cost no more than the time spent hoeing and watering. Our generation is missing this basic staple of self-sufficiency.

At present, approximately 2 percent of our population grows the food that feeds the other 98 percent. Doing it this way has left us in a state of dependency. We've made it the food industry's responsibility to feed us. As a result, most of us wouldn't have the slightest idea how to obtain enough food for ourselves if we ever had to do so, and that leaves us vulnerable.

I don't mean to sound like a conspiracy theorist. I don't believe that our society is about to collapse around us, or that we're all in imminent danger of starvation. But history shows that, over the long term, the fortunes of families, neighborhoods, and nations are never certain. As a complement to the food security afforded us by access to a global food system, local food self-sufficiency is just one more way to build resilience into a community. We may not need it during this generation, or the next, but do we really want that knowledge to pass out of our society?

It's an ignorance we can't afford, not just because it puts future generations at risk if anything happens to our dependable food supply, but because it has also led us to a disconnect from nature and a profound ignorance about living things.

Agrarian knowledge refers to the skills, information, values, and wisdom required to grow food. If we hold these realms of knowledge safe within our communities, pass them along from one generation to the next, as every generation did until the present one, then no matter what uncertainties fate has in store for our progeny, they will always be able to dig a garden, raise up a few plants from seed, and provide themselves with a little sustenance.

There's no way for our society to move away from its addiction to industrial food if we depend on 2 percent of the population to feed the rest of us. The only way that so few can feed so many is through a system of mass production, mass automation, high external inputs, and heavy infrastructure. While acknowledging the benefits of having super-reliable, super-abundant food, throughout the book, we've talked about the environmental, economic, societal, and health problems this system has caused. But the only alternative we can envision at the moment is to exchange mass production for smaller-scale production, to replace at least some of the automation with human labor, and some of the fossil-fuel power with human-muscle power.

In other words, more of us would have to become farmers.

Maybe not dusk-to-dawn, seven-days-a-week farmers, but more of us would need to get back into the business of growing a little bit of our own food.

Whenever we come to the decision that we need to make a change, we tend to assume that this means giving something up. But taking on gardening is a change that gives something back. It adds value to your life in all kinds of unexpected ways. At this moment, you may be wondering how you will fit this new venture into your already jam-packed life, or how you will handle the ickiness of putting your hands in the dirt. But you'll just have to trust me on this: you will never regret the time you spend growing your garden.

Backyard, Balcony, or Kitchen Window?
Where to Plant Your Garden

You need surprisingly little space to grow vegetables. If all you have is a sunny windowsill, you can stick a few pots on it and grow at least something. A couple of herb pots in a window are not going to significantly contribute to your weekly food stocks, but they will help you cultivate your food-growing skills.

Of course, if you have any outdoor space at all, you can do even more. A balcony that gets a few hours of direct sunshine can become home to potted dwarf fruit trees and planter tubs full of vegetables. If you have a postage-stamp-sized yard you can grow a surprising amount of food. A typical suburban half-acre lot, if it gets a lot of direct sun, can grow most of the vegetables your family will need.

What Will You Plant?

If you've never grown anything before, starting a vegetable garden can seem like a daunting task. In an attempt to demystify the process, I asked certified arborist J. D. Willoughby for her advice to first-timers. She recommends starting with a few native plants: "Most of them are easy to grow and very forgiving when it comes to care." She chooses native varieties whose flowers are attractive to bees, and she intersperses them with domestic (non-native)

Top Ten Starter Veggies for Novice Gardeners

Carrots
Garlic
Green beans
Onions
Peas
Peppers
Potatoes
Radishes
Squash
Tomatoes

USDA Plant Hardiness Zones

The USDA identifies eight hardiness zones within the continental U.S. These zones help gardeners determine what to plant and when. See the interactive map at http://plianthardiness.ars.usda.gov.

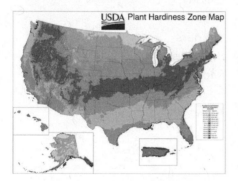

fruit and vegetable plants. "I've found that I get much better pollination on tomatoes, peppers, squash, and pumpkins when I plant flowers and trees that attract pollinators," she said.

Any fruit or vegetable plant that produces a scented flower will need the pollination services provided by bees, so J. D. plants the native varieties that bees find irresistible. "Bee balm (*Monarda didyma* or *Monarda fistulosa*) is probably one of my favorites because it's so easy to grow, very hardy, and does just what it says. It attracts bees—lots of kinds. I also like black-eyed Susans (*Rudbeckia hirta*) and purple coneflower (*Echinacea purpurea*). All three are easy to grow," she said.

I asked J. D. which fruits and vegetables were easiest for first-time gardeners. "Raspberries are very easy to grow," she explained, "and they're usually very productive." She also recommended radishes, garlic, potatoes, and squash.

As you're planning your garden, you might want to consider picking heirloom varieties of fruits and vegetables. Kathy McFarland of Baker Creek Heirloom Seeds said even many experienced gardeners are switching from hybrids to homegrown varieties because they taste better, and because the seeds can be saved and replanted year after year. "Seeds of heirloom varieties will grow to be true to the same kind of plant as the parent, whereas hybrid and genetically modified seeds usually revert to one parent type or the other without consistency," she said. Kathy recommends growing heirlooms to keep these marvelous varieties from going extinct, and to preserve true genetic diversity among domestic species. As to which of the thousands of varieties a home gardener might choose, Kathy advised, "Plant the foods your family likes to eat, start small so as to not become overwhelmed, try new things, keep good records of success and failure, and have fun with it all."

Where to Plant

If you're like me, your first vision of your new vegetable garden probably featured organized rows and squares of plants growing in tidy uniformity. Arborist J. D. Willoughby explained that, although this kind of arrangement may look orderly, your garden will be healthier if you mimic the way Mother Nature plants things. "Nature is messy," she explained. "Not all plants need to grow in neat little rows." She advocates planting flowers among vegetables to attract pollinators and planting different varieties together—partly because it confuses garden pests, but also because companion species can help each other out. She's fond of the Native Americans' "Three Sisters" method of planting corn with beans and squash. Beans use the corn stalks as climbing poles, corn draws from the nitrogen that beans add to the soil, and squash shades the soil to keep down weeds and hold in moisture.

When to Plant

Avid gardeners recognize as many as four growing seasons, depending on their region of the United States. What makes up a growing season in a given region is a combination of average rainfall, available sunlight, and especially, temperature. The USDA identifies eight different hardiness zones in the continental U.S. by their average dates of last frosts and first frosts for the season.

Gardeners usually plant spring gardens as soon as the weather warms a bit, often a month before the last average frost date for their area. The best vegetables to plant in spring are the ones that prefer cool weather and don't mind a light frost. Lettuce, spinach, broccoli, kale, celery, cabbage, peas, bok choi, onions, carrots, potatoes, strawberries, and radishes thrive in a cool spring garden. Don't dump all your seeds into the soil at the same time. Instead, plan successive sowings every two weeks so that you get several progressive harvests instead of a flood.

Warm weather vegetables are sensitive to cold and have to wait until the soil has warmed and danger of frost has passed. After the last frost date for your zone, you can plant tomatoes, peppers, eggplant, cucumbers, squashes, beans, and corn.

Fall gardens are usually planted once the summer veggies have wound down for the season, typically a month before the first frost date for your region. Fall gardens look similar to those of spring: Lettuce, spinach, broccoli, kale, celery, cabbage, bok choi, onions, and carrots, plus parsnips and rutabagas, which are traditionally reserved for fall. As the fall crops grow, the final summer harvests are still coming in: apples, winter squashes, and potatoes.

If you just can't bear to see the growing season come to an end, you can do a few things to extend it. In most moderate growing zones, a polytunnel or hoop house—a long, ribbed tunnel covered in clear plastic—can raise the air temperature under it enough to allow certain cold-hardy plants to grow all winter.

First and Last Frost Dates for USDA Hardiness Zones

First and last frost dates for agricultural hardiness zones. Hardy fruits and vegetables can survive planting a few weeks before last frost. Warm weather plants must wait until after the last frost. Most seed packets will indicate when it's safe to plant.

Zone	Avg Last Frost	Avg First Frost
3	May 15	Aug 15
4	May 15	Sep 15
5	Apr 15	Sep 15
6	Apr 15	Oct 15
7	Apr 15	Oct 15
8	March 15	Oct 15
9	Feb 15	Nov 15
10	Jan 31	Dec 15
11	none	none

In winter, gardeners usually clean up from the year's growing, plant garlic to overwinter, and once the coldest weather sets in, prune their fruit trees. In zones five and southward, gardens can keep producing a few hardy crops outdoors throughout the winter. But even in the coldest zones, anyone with a sunny windowsill can grow a few salad sprouts and a little fresh baby lettuce in the winter months.

Starting Seeds Indoors

Most seed packets come with instructions that tell you whether this particular vegetable can be started indoors for outdoor transplanting later. Typically, the time to start seeds indoors is two weeks before the last frost of the spring for your region. The last frost occurs as late as June 30 for northernmost and mountainous regions, between April 1 and May 30 for the middle of the United States, between March 1 and March 30 for most of California and the South, and February 1 to February 28 in most of Florida and the Gulf Coast.

Take a few cardboard egg cartons and separate the tops from the bottoms. Punch a large hole in the bottom of each egg compartment with a pencil and fill them all with organic potting soil. Press a hole into the center of each bit of soil to the planting depth called for on the seed packet, usually between an eighth and a half of an inch. Tuck in the seed and cover it with soil, then water thoroughly. Plants that have very thick seeds, such as beans, peas, and rhubarb, benefit from soaking for an hour or two before planting. Keep the soil moist. Your seedlings will sprout within a week.

Once they've sprouted, keep your seedlings near a light source. A sunny window is best if you have one; a bright fluorescent light will work if you don't. When the last frost date for your region has passed, you can gently ease your seedling, soil and all, out of its egg compartment and place it in a shallow hole in your garden. Water it thoroughly on planting day.

Making Room for a Mini-Orchard

If you have more than a few square yards of sunny space on your property, odds are you have room for an orchard. Apples, oranges, lemons, limes, grapefruit, pears, peaches, plums, cherries, almonds, avocados, pecans, and hazelnuts all come from trees that can be grown in smallish backyards.

Five Foods You Can Grow Indoors in Winter

Baby lettuce
Baby spinach
Button mushrooms
Radish sprouts
Wheatgrass for juicing

Most of these fruit and nut trees are available in dwarf varieties for supersmall spaces, and some can adapt well to life in a container. As with the rest of your garden family, you'll need to do a little research to see what will grow in your area. Citrus fruits, avocados, walnuts, almonds, and pecans generally don't do well any further north than zone eight. If you live in a zone that's too cold for these tropical and semitropical trees, you might still be able to grow a few of them indoors as long as you have a sunny, humid space that stays warm consistently. Many semitropical fruit and nut trees come in varieties bred to handle indoor life in a pot.

Raspberries, blackberries, and blueberries grow on small bushes. You might have room for a few of these even if fruit trees are impractical for your space. Grapes grow on vines, which can be trained on a trellis placed against a wall.

Keeping Your Soil Healthy

I had an *aha* moment one day when I was turning the soil in my asparagus bed. As I stood catching my breath, looking down at this mysterious, peaty, chocolate-brown substance, I suddenly got it. Those complex, tiny organisms I can't even see are *responsible for my life!* Without them, the plants I depend on wouldn't grow. I live because those plants live. Those plants live because those tiny soil creatures live. At that moment, I felt a connection to life. I knew, deeper than any book-knowing or word-knowing, that I am a living part of this living world. I was overwhelmed with gratitude and belonging.

To anyone who doesn't garden, it's probably difficult to get in touch with this reverence for dirt. But every gardener and farmer I've spoken to says this is what it's all about.

I'm only beginning to understand the basics, but I learned very quickly that soil is healthiest when things are growing in it. That is why many farmers plant cover crops when the harvest is done, so that the soil is always full of life. Because different plant families use nutrients differently, it's also a good idea to rotate what you plant from year to year, so that the soil doesn't get depleted of one particular kind of nutrient. Certain plants also return nutrients to the soil; for instance, peas and beans add nitrogen.

One thing I've had to unlearn about soil is the part about moving it around. Any home improvement store has so many rows of shiny tools perfectly designed for digging into the soil, I thought, surely, that's what you're

Wondrous Variety in Small Suburban Spaces

I live on less than three-fourths of an acre in a suburban neighborhood, and most of my yard is either too shady to grow anything or dominated by a monster septic system. In spite of the modest size of my growing area, and my relative inexperience as a gardener, I've been able to grow a pretty large variety of fruits and vegetables. What follows is an exhaustive list of everything I was able to grow in my yard in just one year:

Asparagus
Basil
Beefsteak tomatoes
Black table grapes
Black walnuts
Bok choi
Broccoli
Butternut squash
Carrots
Celery
Chocolate mint
Chokecherries
Cilantro
Corn
Cucumbers
Dill
Endive
Fennel
Five-color chard
Garlic …

supposed to do with it. But I'm slowly finding out that soil moved is soil *depleted*. The more it's disturbed, the more of its goodness it loses.

For this reason, many gardeners, particularly permaculturists, prefer growing perennials, the kind of plants that don't require replanting. Most of the garden plants we're used to are annuals, meaning you have to keep planting them every year. But some of the most wonderful vegetables are perennials. You can plant them once and they'll keep coming back.

Asparagus, artichokes, and rhubarb are recognized and grown as perennials. But other plants that are often treated as annuals can be encouraged to make an encore appearance. The celery and strawberries in my garden are going on their third year. Fruit and nut trees and berry bushes are great perennial choices, if you have room for them, because you only need to disturb the soil once, on the day you plant them.

Even for annual gardens, there are ways to avoid disturbing the soil. "Many farmers are going to no-till methods, and I think it's an interesting thing for home gardeners to try, too. It certainly saves time," J. D. Willoughby told me. "But you might find that your soil is simply too clayey or has some other issue that might require light tilling. If soil is clayey, don't add sand. Instead, add compost. Rakes are excellent tools and might be a less destructive way to get some soil aeration."

Plant Parenthood: Watering, Weeding, Fertilizing, and Mulching

Your garden probably won't be massively time-consuming, but it will require your attention on a regular basis.

You'll need to check the soil every few days and water whenever it's dry. In hot weather, check it daily. Be careful not to overwater squashes and tomatoes.

After seeing rain barrels on the sides of neighbors' houses, I asked arborist J. D. Willoughby about harvesting rainwater for the garden. "Rain barrels are great for saving water during drought times," she told me, although she noted that collecting and storing rainwater is not legal in all states.

She advised gardeners to first verify that it's allowed in their state, and then "set up barrels so they collect directly from a downspout and then direct the overflow to a garden that can handle being wet for short periods of time. Barrels will fill pretty quickly. A one-inch rainstorm on a 1,000 square foot roof produces more than six hundred gallons of rainwater. Typical barrels have the capacity of about fifty to sixty gallons. And if you collect all that water, you'll need a spectacularly huge garden to use it all before the next storm. One or two barrels should do for most garden needs."

Keep weeds in check. Pull them out when the soil is wet. It's easiest then. Get them when they're small. After your seeds have sprouted, add a layer of mulch. Better yet, grow broad-leafed plants and varieties that create ground cover to discourage weeds.

If you add a lot of great compost to your garden before planting season, you'll only need to fertilize every other week or two. You can buy a good organic fertilizer at most garden shops and mix it with your plant's water, or you can do a little research and make your own homemade organic plant food.

Your garden will thrive better if you keep the soil covered in a layer of mulch. This stuff retains moisture and deters weeds and pests. In cool weather, it also helps insulate your plants and protect them from frost damage.

Getting Rid of What Bugs You

Sooner or later, your plants are going to run into trouble from bugs, molds, fungi, rodents, or any number of other predators. If you're committed to keeping your garden organic, you can find a number of nonsynthetic pesticides at your local garden shop. Or you can try concocting your own. Many organic gardeners swear by sprays made of dish soap, garlic juice, or hot pepper juice.

Some plants are naturally pest-repellant. Many bugs hate the scent of onions and garlic, so some gardeners plant borders of them around their gardens. This past season, I tried planting nasturtiums with my beans and corn and marigolds with my tomatoes. According to garden lore, bugs find both these flowers unbearably stinky. None of the squares where I'd planted them had much trouble with pests.

To stay one step ahead of pests, arborist J. D. Willoughby advocates getting away from the "row" concept of gardens and moving to mixed, diversified plantings. "One thing I've found is that as you increase the diversity in the garden, there are fewer pest problems," she said. "Mix in some flowers with the chives and tomatoes. Scatter the tomatoes in different beds. If you grow ten rows of peppers all together, expect some of them to get pests. It's like a smorgasbord, and the bugs don't have to go very far to eat. But if you scatter

… Grape tomatoes
Golden Delicious apples
Green bell peppers
Green romaine lettuce
Hops
Oak leaf lettuce
Peas
Pumpkins
Radishes
Red cabbage
Red Delicious apples
Red onions
Red peppers
Red raspberries
Red romaine lettuce
Red sails lettuce
Rhubarb
Rosemary
Russian red kale
Strawberries
Virginia peanuts
White onions
Zucchini

the plants around the garden, the pests have to search them out and deal with predators. It makes for a jumbled harvest, but in all, it's a healthier garden."

Harvesting and Storing Your Bounty

Whether you gather it in all at once or cut-and-come-again depends on the types of vegetables you've planted. Anything leafy can usually be lightly snipped and allowed to grow back. Similarly, broccoli will sometimes allow you a second harvest if you cut off the flower heads and let the leaves and stems remain. Savvy gardeners claim that morning is the best time to harvest leafy veggies, because the plant has stored up moisture overnight.

Tomatoes, squashes, peppers, eggplant, and nearly any kind of fruit has to reach a certain level of ripeness before it can be picked. As soon as a tomato starts to change color, you can pick it and place it on a sunny windowsill, and it will continue to ripen, although it will taste best if allowed to ripen on the vine. Squashes will generally do this, too.

Some of your garden bounty will keep in its natural state for an incredibly long time: apples, potatoes, cabbages, and winter squash can sit happily in a cool garage, basement, or enclosed porch for several months, provided they're not exposed to freezing temperatures. Carrots will keep a while if you pack them in a box with sand. Onions and garlic, if you let them grow until their foliage withers and you dry them in the sun for a few days after harvesting, will store well in a kitchen basket for a month or two.

You can also freeze most of your harvest in plastic zip bags or lidded containers. Most vegetables don't freeze well unless you boil or sauté them first. If you have a food processor, you can boil and purée tomatoes, potatoes, and squash for sauces and soups.

The veggies that keep the shortest amount of time are the leafy ones: lettuce, spinach, and kale need to be eaten within a couple days of harvesting. This is why it's an especially good idea to stagger your harvest, so you don't end up with more of these things than you know what to do with.

What About Animals? Raising Chickens, Goats, Bees, and More

I can't speak directly about any of these ventures because I have yet to try them. I want to do them all, but we're not in a location that's zoned for it.

Five Omega-3-Rich Foods You Can Grow at Home

Radish sprouts: 3,358 milligrams
Basil: 2,747 mg
Oregano: 2,732 mg
Marjoram: 2,384 mg
Spinach: 2,183 mg

I've spoken to, and visited with, local people who have raised animals on small amounts of land, and they all recommend it.

A backyard flock of chickens can do much more for you than just give you eggs. They'll dispose of your kitchen scraps, manufacture great manure for your garden, rid your yard of bugs, and mow your lawn. Yes, you read that right. Many backyard poultry enthusiasts build for their birds a contraption known as a chicken tractor: a small enclosed chicken yard, with attached coop, on wheels. The chickens will pick out the bugs lurking in the grass, and they will also keep the grass nicely trimmed and trampled. The tractor is moved to a different spot every few days so that the birds always have a fresh patch of yard to munch on.

I've been enamored of goats for a long time. Years ago, when I lived on a little acreage, I nearly bought two Boer goats to start a dairy herd. I had this idea that keeping animals for milking instead of meat meant I'd never have to slaughter them. It turns out, I wasn't being terribly realistic. In order to produce milk, a goat, cow, or sheep has to produce babies. Of course, I know I'd fall in love with each and every one of them and want to keep them all, and that's how I'd get into trouble. If you're like me, and you're not sure you could slaughter any of your animals when the herd got too numerous, you probably want to leave the raising of the hooved folk to another farmer.

As you've probably read, the world is in need of more hobbyist beekeepers, because we're losing our honeybees. Colony collapse disorder, pesticide use, and other problems are causing them to die by the millions. Backyard beekeeping helps to offset this loss. Every beekeeper I've met speaks lovingly of these amazing insects. A well-tended hive can provide you with two harvests of honey per year, and the rest of the garden benefits from their pollination services.

What Your Garden Will Teach You

Like most things in life that don't involve electronics, growing a garden pays unexpected dividends. In many ways, it's the antidote to modern life. Case in point: attention spans. So much in our modern world keeps our focus shallow and our attention divided. But gardening is so absorbing that it takes the whole of your concentration. When I'm with my plants, I'm more deeply in the moment than at any other time. I am wholly present. My senses open wide. My thoughts flow freely. I'm at peace.

Growing a garden gets you off your tuchis and moving around outdoors. It also does to your soul what a good tune-up does to your car's engine. It does this, first and foremost, by reconnecting you to nature. We're always experiencing the world through eyes and ears, but in your garden, it also comes to you through your nose and knees, your pores and fingernails. You won't just be reading about the life cycles of growing things and the interwoven fabric of soil, air, and weather, you'll be living it, participating in it, and helping it happen.

My garden is teaching me humility. In our society, we've become so self-congratulatory with our limited understanding of nature that we think we can control it. My garden taught me very quickly that nature plays by its own rules. I can knock myself out trying to grow peppers in March or to keep my tomato plants producing in November, but if I'm in the wrong hardiness zone, it ain't happenin'.

My garden is teaching me patience. I can't rush the sprouting of seeds or the ripening of fruit. I can't make the weather warmer or the soil drier. I can only wait until the time is right.

My garden is forcing me to learn to deal with frustrations and disappointments. Sometimes deer will eat every last apple off our trees the night before I was planning to harvest them.

My garden brings me fully into the moment. I can't predict the sudden moments of rapture that come upon me when I'm out there. I look up at just the right moment to see twin monarch butterflies touch down on a leaf in perfect formation. V's of geese fly overhead, morning sun lights up the inside of an unfurling squash blossom, and a tiny round bird the color of a thunderstorm suddenly perches, bobbing, on a branch right in front of me. Beauty simply comes, unbidden, when I'm not expecting it.

OMG-This-Is-So-Easy Quiche

This is such a great recipe for using up that avalanche of vegetables during gardening season. It works for almost all of them. It helps to sauté the veggies lightly before adding them to the quiche, but it's not absolutely necessary.

2 deep dish pie crusts

14 eggs

6 ounces cubed Cheddar, Muenster, Swiss, Havarti, or Smoked Gouda cheese

2 cups diced vegetables of your choice (mix and match as many kinds as you wish)

pepper and herbs to taste (I'm partial to dill)

Divide the cubed cheese and diced vegetables into two even piles. Place them into the pie crusts. In a bowl, beat seven of the eggs. Add a small splash of milk if you like a really fluffy quiche. Add the pepper and herbs. Pour the eggs into one of the pie crusts. Repeat with the other pie crust. Bake at 350 degrees for about a half-hour or until the centers of the quiches are no longer jiggly. If your family, like mine, consists of insatiable carnivores, you can replace one cup of the vegetables with diced ham, crumbled bacon, or sliced sausage.

12

Adjusting Your Lifestyle

Changes to Your Time, Taste Buds, Wallet, and Waistline

When we show our respect for other living things, they respond with respect for us.
—*Arapaho proverb*

It's 6:20 a.m. and there's not a crumb of bread in the house. The boys get on the bus at 6:45 a.m. What will they do about lunch? I haven't had my coffee yet, and I'm already facing a crisis of epic proportions.

What are my options? We just got a delivery of two full bags of gorgeous fresh local vegetables. I could tell them to pack a bunch of radishes, cucumbers, and zucchinis, along with a handful of fresh cilantro. What? Not teenage boy fare? Okay, then I'll whip up a quick batch of biscuits and they can make sandwiches from those. Let me get out the flour—oh, right. I used the last of it on Saturday.

I grab my keys and drive five minutes down the road to the closest grocery store. *Argh*—they don't open until 7:00 a.m. What *is* open? The gas station? I'm desperate enough to try it.

I make one last dash to the 24-hour convenience store attached to the gas station. Stuff on the shelf here is labeled "bread," but it looks more like a slightly toasted version of what I use to wipe down the counters.

Do I send them off with raw zucchinis and risk them not speaking to me for the rest of the week? Or do I give them this stuff, just this once, so that at least they have something to smear their organic peanut butter on? I grab the bread, pay for it, and lead-foot it back home, feeling like an awful mother and swearing never to do this to them again.

Back home, I hand over the fluffy stuff in its colored plastic wrapper, in just enough time for them to make sandwiches. Ben finds the gas station bread amusing. He bites into a slice and pronounces that it's just like marshmallows, without the marshmallow flavor.

Then I start to evaluate the situation. I just violated so many of my own rules, I feel like a hypocrite. I bought one of the most heavily processed food items in the world, one with zero real nutrition, zero flavor, zero reasons for ingesting it at all. I bought a grocery item for my family from a *gas station*, for heaven's sake. How did I let this happen?

We've been wooed into buying industrial food by the promise of convenience. We've come to believe that our busy lifestyles demand it, and we've simply slipped into the habit. We've come to depend on it.

The food industry tells us it's not really their fault. They were only filling a need. After all, now that most moms and dads work full-time and most families don't have a homemaker at the helm, who's available to make food from scratch?

The processed foods that have been around the longest originated, not in the convenience movement of the 1970s or in the hyper-marketing era that began in the 1990s, but in response to consumers' demands for products with longer shelf lives. The first processed foods were developed in the middle of the twentieth century to reduce losses as a result of spoilage. But today, because of massive marketing efforts, grab-and-go, nuke-and-eat foods have become the norm for us, to the point that we don't even question whether this mode of eating really is more convenient, or whether we're sacrificing more than we want to for the sake of getting our food on the go.

Convenience food wasn't really something we asked for. It was an invention that was marketed to us. They dangled the bait, and we bit.

They didn't just stop at selling us on the convenience of their products, either. They went after our self-image. Today, ad campaigns are routinely built around the message that their product will make us cooler, sexier, and more successful. It's no longer just a quick snack. *It's a quick snack that validates our self-worth*.

We Americans, marinated in advertising as we are, have become used to abdicating our decision-making to marketers. We shouldn't feel bad that we were vulnerable to suggestion; as social animals, we're kind of hardwired to respond to what our group expects of us. We do what we need to do in order to fit in. So if we're repeatedly exposed to a message that says we need a certain thing in order to be more acceptable, we're inclined to believe it.

The problem is that those external forces telling us we need to buy something have their own agenda, and it has nothing to do with what's good for us. With all due respect to the benefits that a commercial economy provides to us, the world of commerce exists not to secure our well-being but to make a profit. So if we're not buying as much of their product as they'd like, they'll do whatever it takes to convince us that we should buy more.

In accepting the marketers' message that we need convenient products, we have given up more than we know. We have sacrificed authentic experiences for synthetic ones.

One of the greatest opportunities the local food movement provides for us is a chance to take back that power and learn to make up our own minds again. But making these choices stick will require a few changes. This chapter highlights some of the adjustments you and your family may go through as you let go of your dependence on industrial food.

You May Go Through Convenience Withdrawal

It's absolutely true that getting whole fresh foods from local sources requires more forethought and planning. For one thing, many of them spoil quickly. You'll have to plan meals so that you eat the most delicate foods first, or boil and freeze what you won't get to before they lose their freshness.

Another consideration is that when you buy real, whole foods, you have to do your own processing. Some meals that are infinitely worth eating require several steps. Bean soup, for instance, is definitely not a last-minute meal.

Some foods are so labor intensive that it doesn't make sense to fix just one meal's worth. You'll find it's more efficient to make several batches at once. Granola, burritos, pies, and casseroles fall into this category. It takes only a little additional time to make an extra batch, so you make two: one for tonight and one to freeze for Wednesday night when you know you'll be too busy to cook.

What industrial eaters do with convenience food, a locavore does with leftovers.

This is the way cooks and homemakers have always done things. The difference is that, today, we have to fit these tasks into a turbocharged twenty-first century lifestyle. We have to apply the time management and multitasking skills we've learned in the workplace to the tasks we face in our kitchens.

Top Ten Ways to Maintain Control Over What You Eat

1. Pack food from home whenever you'll be gone for more than three hours. Never let yourself get so hungry that you have to buy and eat whatever is available. Take healthy, less perishable foods that travel well. Some great options include nuts, dried fruits, apples, carrots, and crusty bread with cheese.

2. Shop for meals and snacks rather than just for general groceries. If you shop for a week's worth of food at a time, buy ingredients for seven breakfasts, lunches, and dinners, plus one or two snacks per day. This way, you'll have enough good stuff on hand, as well as a plan for feeding yourself that will carry you through until the next shopping trip.

3. Assume you're going to be too busy to cook sometimes. On Sunday, cook that night's dinner plus one or two more freezable dinners, so that if you get too busy to cook one night, you can whip out and thaw a home-cooked meal instead of ordering pizza.

4. Make homemade treats on a regular basis. This way, you won't feel deprived of the donuts, chips, and ice cream you used to buy just because they were fun. You and your loved ones deserve to have a treat now and then. Making it at home just doubles the fun.

5. Before you leave for a party, eat a medium-sized meal at home. That way, if all your host has on offer is cocktail weenies and cheese puffs, you can nibble politely so as not to offend, but you won't have to view the buffet table as a source of sustenance.

6. Eat something every three hours so that hunger doesn't make you crazy. When you're so ravenous you could chew your own arm off, you're less likely to make rational decisions about what to eat. You should be a little hungry before a meal, but if you're starting to act like sharks do when they smell chum in the water, you've gone without food a little too long.

7. Eat nutritious meals. Eat a wide variety of fruits, vegetables, and whole grains, foods with a lot of fiber. You will probably find that the more complete your nutrition, the fewer cravings you have.

8. Drink water when you're thirsty. Sometimes thirst seems like hunger. Stay hydrated so that you won't give your body food when what it really needs is water.

9. Get a lot of rest and exercise. Many of us eat because we're tired, or even because we're restless. If, like me, you're in the habit of eating for reasons other than hunger, identify those reasons and give your body what it really needs. If you get eight hours of great sleep a night and at least thirty minutes of exercise a day (which helps with the sleeping), you will be less likely to use food to relieve fatigue and restlessness.

10. Face your pain instead of numbing it with food. Food is so deeply keyed to our sense of survival and well-being that many of us eat it not for nourishment but to comfort ourselves when we're unhappy. The problem with candy bars, donuts, and potato chips is that, especially when you're depressed, stressed, or PMSed, *they really do make you feel better*, at least for the moment. If you're tired, angry, ill, lonely, anxious, or unfulfilled, it will be difficult to avoid using sugary, fatty, salty foods to alleviate your pain. So do yourself a favor and fix what's wrong instead of trying to manage the fallout.

You'll Get Reacquainted With Your Kitchen

There are only two ways to enjoy the benefits of whole, fresh, local foods: cook it yourself, or hire a full-time chef to prepare it for you. Assuming a kitchen staff is not in your budget, this means you and your kitchen will be seeing a lot more of one another.

Now, you and I both know you don't have time to do all that prepping, cooking, and washing up every day. You have a demanding career and many other obligations on your time. You're probably not planning to give up your job to become a full-time homemaker, though I'd applaud you if you did. So how do you manage kitchen duty along with your other responsibilities?

You don't do it alone. You share it with family, friends, and neighbors.

If you live by yourself, you can buddy up with a nearby neighbor who also lives alone to divide up weekly cooking duties: one person cooks for two every other night. As long as both people's food preferences are similar, this works fine. You can also avail yourself of communal meals at clubs and faith groups. One student told me she loves potlucks because they give her an opportunity to cook for others.

The local food movement has the potential to impact American family structure in a powerful way. It's an opportunity to create a more equitable division of labor in the household, as well as a chance to bring the benefits of homemaking back into our lives.

The twentieth century saw enormous changes in domestic roles. Traditionally, household work was accorded to women, people of color, undereducated people, and anyone born into the lowest economic strata. As a result of the civil rights and women's rights movements of the 1960s and 1970s, the workplace opened its doors to a broader segment of society, including the groups who previously had few other options than domestic work.

But even though women and other low-status groups took on new responsibilities in the workplace, they didn't automatically shed their household duties. During the 1980s and 1990s, the mom of the family got double duty. After an eight- or nine-hour shift at the office, Mom had to race home, cook dinner, schlep Ashley and Brittany to piano lessons, and run Jason's bath, while Dad still got to come home to a home-cooked meal and then put his feet up and relax.

In the early part of this century, women have gradually shed the so-called second shift. But Dad didn't move into the kitchen to fill the void. Instead, the family ditched homemaking and got accustomed to convenience foods and takeout meals. Many folks in the local food movement have discovered that when we let go of cooking, we lost more than we bargained for, and they think we need to bring it back.

What if, this time, cooking is not the responsibility of one, but it is spread equally among all members of the family?

If you propose bestowing kitchen duty on your spouse and kids, I can guarantee what their first response will be: *I don't have time!* Since no one has figured out how to grow extra hours in a day, your family will have to work this out. It might be a good idea to make this decision together. What's worth letting go of to free up that extra hour for dinner prep?

Food Will Become an Investment

A similar shift may have to happen to your family budget. Until you get the hang of it, you'll probably be spending more upfront for groceries. You'll feel the sticker shock. You may need significant chunks of cash to buy food in bulk when the opportunity arises, rather than the predictable wad of grocery money you were used to setting aside for the weekly grocery run.

You may also find that you need to invest in a number of tools to build yourself a truly functional kitchen. You'll have to trust that it's far cheaper to live this way than it is to dine on fast food and frozen dinners, and that's even before you factor in what you will save in medical costs over a lifetime of healthier eating.

At first, you'll only be aware of the extra outlay of money upfront. But over time, you'll begin to realize that you're actually *saving* money by eating home-cooked food. If you're like me, you'll discover that you're not spending nearly as much pocket money on junk from convenience stores and vending machines. As you lose your taste for processed food, you'll develop a preference for holding out until you can get home to eat the good stuff. You'll fill a thermos with coffee before you leave home instead of blowing five dollars on a latte. You'll grab a plastic container with last night's casserole and a couple of pieces of fruit on your way out the door in the morning, and save the eight dollars you would have spent on chicken tenders and fries at the lunch counter.

Five Things to Cut Back On to Make Time to Cook

Shopping
Texting
Television
Web surfing
Video games

Your Taste Buds Will Change Allegiance

When we switched from processed, industrial food to fresh, local foods, we were amazed at how quickly our tastes adjusted. Within a few weeks, we began to notice the chemical additives in any processed foods we tasted. We all became much more sensitive to sugar. Foods that had simply tasted sweet to us before now seemed unbearably cloying. Salt began to pack more of a wallop as well. We stopped adding it to dishes we cooked, and we used less of it at the dinner table.

It turns out that, at least in these experiences, we were normal.

Although humans are hardwired to derive pleasure from sweet tastes, the level of sweetness we experience is a matter of comparison. If you're used to drinking orange-flavored drink mix, fresh squeezed orange juice might at first taste metallic and bitter by comparison. But if orange juice is your normal morning beverage, you'll probably find the drink mix overwhelmingly sweet.

As a general rule, humans find tastiest those foods that are familiar to them. Everybody loves sweetness, especially kids, but other taste preferences must be learned. The more times your family is exposed to a particular food, the more acceptable they'll find it. We tend to dislike flavors that are strange to us, and like the taste of the ones that evoke feelings of comfort and safety—in other words, foods we eat at home a lot.

Habits are formed through repetition. Odds are, if you and your family eat fresh local food every day, your taste buds and expectations will adjust, and home-cooked meals will become your new normal.

Your Doctor Might Be Seeing Less of You

Your own body will convince you faster than any medical study. When you eat fresh whole foods, you feel better. Eating local food is a powerful way to take control of your health. You'll probably also find that, with this kind of food, you stay satisfied longer on smaller portions.

Will a diet of fresh local foods make you lose twenty pounds in a month? I wish I could say it will. Unfortunately, it doesn't work that way.

We've been eating mostly local food for nearly two years. My husband has lost twelve pounds. I've lost about eight. I'm nearly as overweight as I was before, but it's not the local food's fault. It's because, even though overall

I'm eating healthier, I still overeat for the worst reasons. I eat whenever I'm lonely, angry, tired, frustrated, or bored. I eat too much of the foods that give me a rush: high fat, crunchy, salty, and sweet. I haven't lost much weight because, although my overall diet has gotten much healthier, I still abuse food in much the same way as I always have. That, plus my ongoing struggle to get up from my desk and move more often, is keeping the pounds on.

You will certainly be healthier than you would be on a diet of junk food, but if you're in the habit, as I am, of frying your local food in oil, slathering it in butter, and topping it with cheese, you'll be just as much at risk for obesity, and for the host of nasty diseases that go along with it. Eating sensibly is still the responsibility of those doing the eating.

So, if you're like me, your overall poundage will stay the same unless you also change your portions and your physical activity level. But you may find that a switch to more whole fresh foods will help you with this. Fresh food is tastier and more filling, so you'll probably find that you can get by on less of it. You may also find that real food gives you more energy, so it may be easier to get up and take that afternoon walk.

Then there are a few intangible health benefits that may come your way. I can't quantify this, but I've noticed that over the past two years we've had far fewer colds, flus, and stomach upsets. We've been less stressed. We've slept better. We've had more energy. I can't draw an unequivocal line between these phenomena and the changes in our diet, but I believe it's had something to do with it.

Your Kids, Garden, and Dog May Be Seeing More of You

One of the most powerful benefits of eating real food is its ability to foster connections—with other humans and with nature.

Earlier in the chapter, I suggested that the way to fit cooking into a busy modern lifestyle is to share kitchen time with loved ones. Any shared activity is likely to draw you closer, but one that produces something wonderful for the whole family to enjoy does it even more so. The consequence is that you may find that your relationships with your spouse and your kids grow deeper.

In a similar vein, as your relationship to real food grows, it can't help but deepen your relationship to nature. If you permit yourself to fall in love with food, not just the stuff that ends up on your plate, but the real, whole

Brew Your Own!

Where my passion for local food has led me into the garden, it's lured my husband, Al, into the basement. That's where, for the past two years, he's been quietly squirreling away the packages that have arrived from home-brewery suppliers. The first few batches of Al's homemade beer were—*ahem*—interesting, but last fall, he poured up a gorgeous, foamy oatmeal stout that rivaled anything our local microbreweries serve.

life form you hold in your hands before it becomes dinner, you'll be drawn into a deeper experience with it. You'll find that you can't recreate the true color of a living thing with any paints humankind has devised. You'll have that mind-blowing *aha*-moment when you realize that nothing in nature is only one color. You discover that every plant, and every *part* of the plant, has a remarkable architecture. You see yourself in that living thing: skin, flesh, veins, cells. It breathes; you breathe. It eats; you eat. It grows; you grow.

If you get this far into your love affair with real food, you're bound to want to grow some of it yourself. That impulse will send you out into the backyard with a shovel. That's when you become a gardener, a person who shepherds life forms through their natural cycles and gets to eat the results.

As you permit yourself to fall in love with nature, you may find you're drawn into newer and deeper interactions with it. The boost in your energy level may make you available to walk your dog more. This daily canine-human bonding ritual, plus your deepening appreciation of nature, may allow you to see your dog in a new light: less as a human accessory, more as a creature in her own right. You may find it easier to appreciate and nurture her essential dog-ness, instead of expecting her to conform to human ways.

What You Ate Before vs. What You'll Eat Now

Before	Now
Sugar	Honey
Soda	Iced tea (*herbal* tea is grown locally everywhere)
Potato chips	Popcorn
Boxed cereals	Homemade granola
Chicken tenders	Whole chicken
Hash brown patties	Baked potatoes
Turkey pot pies	Chicken stew
Mac and cheese	Squash casserole (don't knock it 'til you try it)
Burgers	Chilis

Will You Allow Yourself a Few Meaningful Luxuries?

How strictly you choose to adhere to a local food policy is a matter of individual choice. If your conscience dictates that you never eat a morsel that comes from more than a hundred miles away, you're a braver woman or man than I.

I don't really want to be a hundred-mile purist. It's hard to imagine a lifetime without *any* imported food. In all likelihood, this would mean never again tasting cinnamon, nutmeg, bananas, chocolate, or coffee. I'm getting depressed just thinking about it. Could we allow for a few exceptions to the rule, so long as we choose local options as often as it makes sense to do so?

You'll probably find it easier to make a long-term commitment to sustainable eating if you permit yourself a few caveats and occasional splurges. I hope I've made the case by now that I'm not anti-industrial food. I'm not going to suggest that you boycott grocery stores. I think of this change as a process. If, day to day, you're *mostly* making choices that move you toward a more healthful, sustainable way of life, that's real progress.

Can You Dine Out and Still Eat Local?

If you enjoy dining out, but you don't want to utterly abandon your commitment to local food every time you treat the family to a night on the town, you do have options. Today, many restaurants, from fancy to family-friendly, are getting into the local food movement. Those establishments that serve local foods, often referred to as "farm to table" restaurants, often include a statement to that effect in their advertisements. To find restaurants in your area that incorporate local foods into their menus, visit www.dinegreen.com and plug in your state, or go to www.eatlocalgrown.com and plug in your zip code.

But suppose you're on the road and you don't have the means to look up the nearest local-food-based restaurant. If you have to wing it, choose family-owned restaurants rather than franchises. Try to avoid chain restaurants, especially of the fast food variety, because they're unlikely to have anything nonindustrial on their menus. When dining out, I try to avoid ordering meat. Unless the menu specifies otherwise, it's likely to have come from a CAFO. One local restaurant stated proudly on its menu that its burgers were made from *100 percent corn-fed beef!* Either the chefs themselves were ignorant, or they were betting on the ignorance of their diners. If I go with a vegetarian dish, I may not be eating local, but at least I'm avoiding the worst of the industrial food system.

Food Will Move to the Center of Your Family's Life

As you move deeper into a deliberate relationship with food, you'll find that it has taken up residence at the center of your life. Historically, this is the normal place for it. The majority of human activity has been focused on obtaining, preparing, and eating food.

Food will form the rationale behind the work you do as a family: snapping green beans, baking cookies, shucking corn. All these tasks give you a reason to spend meaningful time together.

Food also becomes a means of entertainment, of spending leisure time in a fun and productive way. Quiet vacation days, rainy days, and snow days become opportunities to play around in the kitchen, time to test out new recipes.

My son Phillip has taken on a number of culinary adventures, including his hot chili pepper experiment. He'd read about the Scoville scale that ranks

Fireside Friday at Black Ankle Vineyards: An Hour of Sustainable Happiness

Our car climbs through night forest on a narrow, winding paved road. We turn at the Black Ankle sign and dip suddenly onto a steep track twisting through the vineyard toward the yellow lights of the lodge. Arched doorway. Broad wooden beams. Logs smolder on the stone hearth. Candles shudder in the puff of cold air we let in as we enter. A curly haired musician strums an acoustic guitar in one corner.

Every inch of this place is deliberate. I run my hand over the marble smoothness of the bar that was pressed from the branches of the first vines planted here. We order a bottle of red wine that was grown, made, and bottled here. It has never left home. We select a freshly baked baguette and a wheel of creamy goat cheese from a Maryland dairy.

We set our wine down carefully. The tables are carved from polished slabs of trees. Gaps yawn in the surface, large enough to swallow up a misplaced bottle. We slice into hot bread and velvet cheese. In the candlelight, we catch one another's eyes. The guitar player strums softly. We pour the wine: smoky and spicy, and dark. A wine full of secrets. We savor the bread and cheese: creamy-sharp, salty-sweet.

In this place, everything—the food, the architecture, even the music—is made by hand, locally, with love.

The wine writes a novel on my tongue. We empty the bottle of its last ruby-red drop and smear the last of the cheese on the heel of the bread. The evening steals away. The youngster with the guitar strums the last few notes, packs up his instrument, slips on his coat, and heads for home. Then, warmed and deeply contented, we do the same.

---

the "heat" of peppers, from zero for a sweet bell pepper to two million for the Trinidad Moruga Scorpion. Last August, he procured about a dozen peppers of different Scoville ratings, sat down at the kitchen table with a glass of milk for putting out the fire, and set himself the task of tasting each pepper, from sweetest to hottest. In the interest of science, he videotaped his reaction to each one. Always the supportive family, we stood dutifully by and laughed our butts off. I screwed up my courage and tasted a bhut jolokia pepper, clocking in at more than a million on the Scoville scale, but only after Phillip had pronounced it survivable. It felt just like a wasp sting on my tongue.

Food will provide your family with learning opportunities. Visiting a farm or working in the garden is a chance to learn the ways of nature. Shopping at farmers' markets is an opportunity to learn about economics. The kitchen brings opportunities for lessons in everything from chemistry to culture.

For millennia, families have worked and laughed together over the collecting and preparing of food, and a good meal has always been at the center of any gathering of loved ones. In bringing food to the heart of your family's life, you've returned it to its normal place.

Food Truck Fans Rejoice! Local Food on Wheels

You might not expect to find local food served from the window of a food truck, but if you're around Wellfleet, Mass., this summer, you're in for a treat. J'aime and Christian Sparrow have been specializing in offering dishes made with local provender from their truck, Sunbird, since 2012. Their menu features items whose ingredients are 50 percent to 70 percent local, obtained from a dozen nearby farms.

I asked J'aime how they came to the decision to offer local foods from their truck. She told me, "We grew up in the restaurant business in San Francisco where fantastic local products are available year-round. For us, there really is no other way to eat and be a part of a community. We wanted to share that lifestyle with visitors, neighbors, and friends."

Offering local foods from a truck presents unique challenges. "In the restaurant business, consistency is superimportant," J'aime said. "The goal of most traditional food businesses has been to create semistatic menus that guests come to know and depend on. This requires having access to the same ingredients time and again. In contrast, when you buy food locally, you quickly find that small crops, grown close by, are not always available or consistent." J'aime and Christian meet this challenge with creativity, flexibility, and inspiration. They nurture a healthy respect for seasonal eating. "If one thing is not available, then another might be," J'aime said. "It inspires us to come up with a new menu item on the fly."

J'aime and Christian adjust their cooking methods to suit the seasonal changes in food items. "In the spring," J'aime explained, "pea sprouts are tender and delicious. They make great additions to salads and can be sautéed on their own with a little butter and sea salt. As the plants mature, the focus shifts to the actual peas themselves. There is very little you have to do to a garden pea, picked at its peak, to make it yummy. Then, as their season fades, peas become a bit more woody and fibrous. You don't have to give up on them. Simmer them with some onions, carrots, and herbs to make a tasty broth that can then be used in a late-summer garden vegetable soup."

The higher upfront cost of local foods also presents some challenges. J'aime and Christian understand the reasons small producers have to charge more. "As purveyors of these products, we walk a fine line between sustaining our business and providing a great product at a fair price," J'aime said. "We make the most of each item when it's in season, and develop recipes with very little waste. That way, we can spend a little more on the food we serve, charge enough to stay in business, and avoid alienating our customers with outrageous prices."

I asked J'aime how customers respond to their local food specialties. "People are genuinely excited and curious about our products, processes, and the local growers and catchers that we are associated with," she said. "Not only is local food sustenance for the person eating it, it's a way of connecting the dots in their community in a very intimate way. Growers, purveyors and consumers are directly linked to one another, to the land, the sea, the produce, and the animals they provide for our survival."

Even though they're fully aware of the social, economic, and environmental importance of their contribution, these two food pros are not about to let the mood get too heavy. "There are a lot of folks out there who just want to eat good food and relax," J'aime said. "It doesn't always have to be a statement. Enjoying good food is just … good."

Stuffed Roasted Rosemary Chicken With Portobella Mushrooms and Potatoes

My son Phillip developed this recipe after he discovered how much he liked mushrooms.

1 pastured roasting chicken

8 small red-skinned potatoes, diced into large pieces

4 portobella mushrooms, diced into large pieces

1 cup olive oil

4 cloves garlic, sliced

2 sprigs fresh or dried rosemary, crumbled (about a tablespoon)

Sea salt (optional)

Par-boil the potatoes and cut them in half. Rinse the chicken thoroughly and pull out whatever's inside its body cavity. Place the bird breast-upward on a rack inside a roasting pan.

Fry the potatoes with the garlic and half the rosemary in oil on high heat until the potatoes are golden, then reduce the heat to medium and add the portobellos. Fry briefly. Stuff the potato-mushroom-garlic-rosemary mixture into the chicken. Drizzle the chicken with olive oil. Sprinkle the remaining rosemary over the chicken. Sprinkle with salt, if desired.

Roast the chicken at 375 degrees for about an hour and a half, or until it's golden brown and the meat is no longer pink inside. Phillip has been known to serve this meal with side dishes of carrots, Swiss chard, and apple biscuits. This kid can cook!

Part 4

How Local Eating Affects Your World

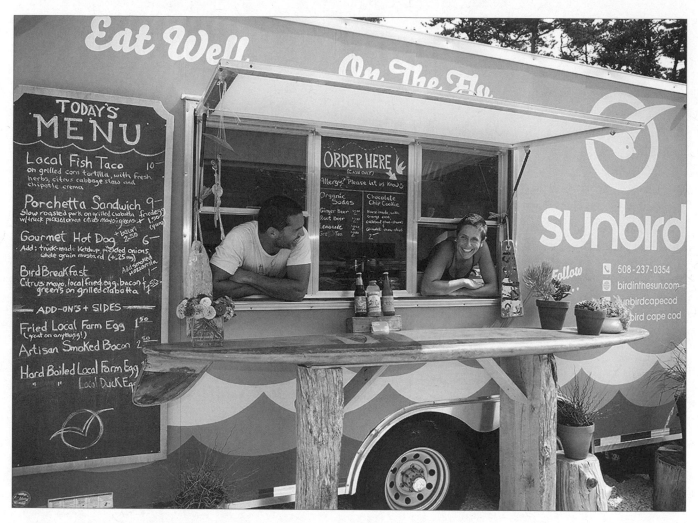

The Sunbird food truck serves local food at the beach (see page 205)

13

Fostering Connections

How Local Food Supports Families and Communities

The strength of a nation derives from the integrity of the home. —*Confucius*

One day last summer, when I was cleaning up after class, I heard a knock on my classroom door. Through the door's small window, I saw a woman I didn't know holding up two plates of blue-and-white-frosted chocolate birthday cake and smiling broadly.

I opened the door, and still smiling, she said, "You don't know me, but my department was celebrating a birthday and we had all this leftover cake. I grew up in the South, and I was raised with the idea that if you had food, you shared it. So I decided, instead of throwing away this extra cake, I would see if I could find a good home for it. Would you like some?"

I accepted the smaller of the two pieces and thanked her.

She grinned even wider and said, "I feel like I just connected with my roots. Thank you for letting me honor a fine tradition!"

The cake she gave brought me pleasure for a couple of seconds. But the smile on her face as she shared food with a stranger will stay with me for a long time.

This brief encounter left me deeply aware of the power that food has to connect us. Eating is not just a mechanical act. It can also be a shared experience, and an occasion for reaching out to people.

In recent decades, we've moved away from a lifestyle conducive to sharing food. Sociologist Robert Putnam, in his book *Bowling Alone: The Collapse and Revival of American Community*, reports that the number of families who claim that they regularly eat dinner together has declined in the last twenty years to 34 percent. As communities abdicate more of their food production to large, distant corporations, food-sharing activities that were once the hub of community life—potluck suppers, community picnics, having friends over for dinner—seem to have faded in importance.

Bringing real, whole food back into our lives creates an opportunity to rebuild the connections we lost when we ceded control of our food lives to big business. Local food requires a return to the concept of meals, which is a return to the concept of sharing.

In this chapter, I'll frame the shared meal as a quintessential human bonding experience. I'll discuss how an intimate relationship with food—growing it, preparing it, cooking it, and sharing it with loved ones—builds character and strengthens families. I'll show how choosing local food enhances communities and bolsters local economies. And I'll throw out a few random ideas I've had about the entrepreneurial opportunities a local food economy might create.

The Anthropology of the Shared Meal

Sitting down to a meal with loved ones is an activity that predates our species. The earliest members of our genus, *homo*, were cooperative hunter-gatherers dependent on membership in small groups. The lives of the few hunter-gatherers left today give us a glimpse into this lifestyle. Foraging people share food communally, usually through a system of rules that dictate how food is to be distributed. Since the advent of farming, the rules surrounding the sharing of food have grown more complex, but the value of eating as a shared experience has remained the norm throughout human history.

When we modern Americans began to abandon shared meals in order to accommodate hectic lifestyles and asynchronous schedules, we may have given up more than we realized. Shared meals strengthen the bonds between people, build group identity, create shared memories, and teach a "grammar" of civility and cooperation.

Food as Gift Predates Food as Commodity

For the vast majority of the time our species has lived on this planet, food was not a thing to be bought and sold, but a community resource to be shared among all members of the group. Even today, many traditional people follow powerful rules that govern the sharing of food.

Reciprocity

Giving and taking without the use of money.

Commodity

An item that is bought and sold.

Long before the advent of money, when people lived in groups small enough that each member could count everyone else as a relative, people met one another's needs through a system known as reciprocity. Reciprocity between close relations amounted to doing a good turn for one another. You do for your kinsman with the understanding that he would do the same for you as the need arose.

Even in a complex post-industrial civilization like ours, we still use this system with our closest family members and friends. In fact, reciprocity of any kind only works among people who share a relationship, which is why, in a society like ours, where most people are strangers to each other, it can't be the only form of exchange.

Reciprocity among community leaders sometimes amounted to grand giveaways of food and other goods. Anthropologist Andrew Strathern writes in *The Rope of Moka* that the chiefs of the Trobriand Islands near New Guinea would take turns making *moka*, a ceremonial gift-giving event in which one chief would present to another as many pigs as he could possibly afford. The more pigs he gave, the greater his status. The receiver of the gift pigs would then have to outdo the gift by giving even more pigs, if he wished to maintain his dignity. In the meantime, all this pig-giving meant pork dinners for a great number of people, a handy form of economic redistribution.

To an anthropologist, this sort of gift giving creates a bond of obligation between giver and receiver. No cash changes hands in this kind of exchange, because people are motivated by responsibilities to one another rather than personal gain. It's a group-centered rather than ego-centered system.

In pointing out that food was historically shared, I'm not saying we should abandon commerce and try to go back to a system of 100 percent reciprocity. For one thing, it wouldn't work. For another, I'm absolutely in favor of farmers being paid *really well* for the food they grow. But the neat thing about economic systems is that we don't have to choose just one. We can pay for food in the contexts in which it's appropriate—for instance, when we buy food from local farmers who have the specialized knowledge to grow it—but still appreciate the sharing, bonding, and gifting of food within neighborhoods, communities, and families.

I see a benefit in the mind-set that having a lot of food comes with an obligation to share it, especially with those who have less. I hope we decide to hang on to this value, because I want to live in a world where everyone eats well.

Food Among Friends

Like most anthropologists from Western cultures, David Counts of McMaster University had to learn the rules of reciprocity the hard way. In an article published in Philip DeVita's *The Humbled Anthropologist*, Counts wrote that during the first year he lived with his family in the village of Kandoka in Papua New Guinea, he inadvertently offended many of his neighbors—first by offering to pay for a watermelon that the elder insisted should have been a gift and, later, by refusing a gift of bananas from a neighbor when they had far more than they needed. By the end of their stay, they had learned the rules of food-sharing among friends: never pay for a gift of food and never refuse food, even if you have plenty, because having a lot just means you've got more to share with others.

Feed Thy Neighbor: No Pehunan, No War

The Semai people of West Malaysia are known for their strong preference for peace. They're one of a tiny handful of nonviolent human societies. What keeps the Semai peaceful, while most other societies regularly engage in violent conflict? Anthropologist Clayton Robarchek claims that it comes down to the Semai's concept of *pehunan*, a state of want or dissatisfaction a person may experience, which the Semai believe the group is obligated to fulfill. A person in need is a danger, both to himself and the group. It's the obligation of every person in the community to feed, clothe, shelter, and include anyone in a state of *pehunan*. To refuse to do so places the group at risk for conflict. If, as the Semai assert, conflict is a result of unmet needs, then the group must *meet those needs*. They simply don't see violence as an option.

Meals Strengthen Group Identity

Whenever we sit down to a shared meal, we create a shared identity. No human group eats everything that's edible in its environment. Every society has rules about what's good to eat and what's not, and human groups identify themselves, in part, by the foods they eat. My husband, Al, whose family comes from Puerto Rico, tells me it's often said of a child who has the look of someone from the island, "you can see the rice and beans in his face."

In her book *Purity and Danger: An Analysis of Concepts of Pollution and Taboo,* anthropologist Mary Douglas studied the kosher laws practiced by people of the Jewish faith and concluded that, together, they made a statement about "being true to one's kind." She claimed that there were no laws pertaining to plants, because plants don't have behavior. According to kosher rules, a proper land animal walks on cloven hooves and chews its cud, so bats are out because they fly, and dogs and cats are off the menu because they "walk on their hands." Consuming a kosher meal is a deeply symbolic act, both because it makes a statement about the kind of self-discipline required to live a just and holy life, and because it creates a shared identity among the eaters.

Meals Create Shared Memory

In his article "A Tale of Easter Ovens: Food and Collective Memory," published in the Spring 2008 edition of the journal *Social Research,* anthropologist David Sutton writes about the power of food to create "collective memory" within a society. He explains that, on the Greek island of Kalymnos, food is deliberately tied to memory at funerals. Bereaved family members feed *kollivo,* a sweet cake with fruit and nuts, to friends and neighbors, while reciting the phrase "in his memory." Sutton says members of the community share kollivo with all passers-by in the name of the deceased.

Food is so important to the creation of shared memories that, sometimes, people even plan ahead for the remembering they're about to do. Sutton claims that when families prepare for an important meal together, they're engaging in "prospective memory"—planning in the present for future memories, getting themselves ready to remember the meal and how it tasted. Food shared in a ritual context simultaneously constructs and recalls memories, creating continuity with the past.

Meals Create a Grammar of Community

Food that's brought into the home whole and in a relatively natural state, whether bought or harvested, must be carried in, prepared, and cooked. In other words, it demands to be eaten as a meal.

What turns the act of eating into a meal? According to anthropologist Sidney Mintz, a "meal" is a shared experience. Everyone in the group eats it at the same time, usually to the exclusion of other activities. The same choice of foods is shared by all, rather than having each diner select the food he or she prefers. At a meal, portions are communal, too. When a person serves herself from a communal serving plate, she doesn't just take the portion she desires, but adjusts her portion to the needs of the other diners.

In his book *Sweetness and Power*, Mintz explains that a meal has rules and guidelines, in the same way that language has grammar. "We cannot speak without grammar," says Mintz, but "we can eat without meals." We can, and will, go on eating, even if the notion of a "meal" disappears, which is precisely the way our society has been trending over the past few decades.

Eating Christmas

According to anthropologist Richard Borshay Lee, in his essay "Eating Christmas in the Kalahari," the Ju/Wasi, hunter-gatherers of the Kalahari Desert in Africa, first came to know Christmas through British missionaries in the nineteenth century. The centerpiece of Ju/Wasi Christmas is a massive ox roast. For them, as for us, it's a celebration of fellowship, but as Lee discovered, the rules of communal eating take a slightly different form in their society.

One Christmas, Lee went out of his way to select the largest, fattest ox as a gift for his neighbors. But when he told them about it, he was dismayed at their response: "Do you expect us to eat that bag of bones?" They grumbled that he must be blind if he couldn't tell the difference "between a proper cow and an old wreck." Because he had already bought the ox, he had no choice but to butcher it and serve it to his guests on Christmas Day. They feasted, laughed, and danced for two days and nights, and they happily took home the leftovers.

When Lee finally asked his guide for an explanation of this paradox, he was told that the Ju/Wasi never overtly praise a member of their group for his or her contribution, lest that person develop a big ego. In a society without formal means of conflict resolution, conflict is kept at bay by cultural institutions such as this one.

So, if you ever celebrate Christmas in the Kalahari, expect your roast beef dinner to be served up with a heaping helping of humble pie.

Mintz speaks of the decline of the American concept of the meal. He states that food marketers tend to cast the meal in negative terms, as "an obstruction to the exercise of individual preferences," and that the modern habit of combining eating with entertainment and other pleasurable activities, to maximize enjoyment, tends to place the emphasis on consumption. As the availability of an array of food choices has increased, the social nature of the meal has declined.

Convenience Means You Never Have to Share: Values in a Commoditized World

Meals are much more than communal face-stuffings. The act of eating together solidifies bonds, creates identity, builds shared memory, and reinforces the values, attitudes, and behaviors that keep a community together.

Yet, there's something about a highly commoditized market economy that discourages this fundamental sharing of food. In fact, it seems to discourage the sharing of anything at all. The difference between an economic exchange based primarily on reciprocity and one based on commerce is that a commercial exchange tends to be egocentric. It emphasizes individual gain, and each individual is encouraged to focus on gratifying her own needs.

The values in a highly commoditized world, where we're encouraged to meet every need and want by buying something, revolve around the self. We prize standing out, making our mark, outdoing our competition, and defeating our critics. We're viewed as clever and sexy if we can manipulate people into giving us what we want. A society with a highly commercialized economy encourages greed, selfishness, competition, and an expectation that we should get what we want whenever we want it. Just watch ten minutes of TV commercials, and you'll see this message played over and over.

Last summer, out of curiosity, I struck up a conversation on this topic with some of the kids in my enrichment classes. I asked, "What really makes a person happy? Is it getting everything they want?" I expected them to say no, that what made them happiest was their family, their friends, or their pets. Instead, to my astonishment, most of them said yes, that happiness was all about getting what they wanted.

Because studies have determined that the average American kid is exposed to more than twenty thousand advertising messages per year, I suppose this response shouldn't have been too surprising. Especially in the realm of food ads, kids are encouraged to think in terms of personal gratification. Foods aren't marketed to them as nourishment, but as entertainment. I'm thinking about how many kids' cereal ads feature one character trying to filch a meal while other characters try to stop him. If you're picturing certain cartoon rabbits, toucans, and leprechauns, you probably grew up with the same cereal commercials that I did. The selfishness and duplicity with which these characters try to obtain the cereal is about as far as you can get from the value of food as a gift meant to be shared.

If we're not crazy about the values imparted by commercialized food, we do have an alternative. We can return to food as a shared experience. Local food practically demands to be shared. It has little or no advertising. It makes no ridiculous claims. In contrast to mass-produced convenience foods, which are tailored to meet the desires of the self, and require little investment of time, thought, or values, local-sustainable foods are perfect for sharing. By its very nature, food into which someone has invested time and effort creates an occasion for that quintessentially human ritual, the *meal*.

Involvement With Food Brings Kids Back to Reality

During summers, when I teach enrichment classes to kids who range in age from nine to fifteen, I've discovered that there are two distinct groups of students who come into my classes. About one-fourth of the kids have microscopic attention spans. They get bored and frustrated easily. Their interaction with their peers seems to be driven by competition. They're far more likely to be selfish and rude. The artwork they create often depicts scenes of violence.

In contrast, the other group of kids—the majority—can usually entertain themselves quietly while they're waiting for the next task. They're more likely to see difficult activities as challenges and can understand that failures bring learning opportunities. They'd rather cooperate with their peers than compete with them. They express themselves with ample vocabularies. They bring a breadth of knowledge and perspectives to class discussions.

What's the difference between these two groups? What I often discover, after interacting with them for a while, is that the kids with the shortest attention spans and poorest social skills are the ones who have spent a large chunk of their childhood playing video games. The kids with the best attitudes, most creativity, and greatest social skills are the ones who have spent the most time doing real things in the real world, alongside friends and family.

The kids who play a lot of video games are missing out on the experiences that build confidence, teach problem solving, enhance communication skills, and help them cope with frustration. They have fewer interactions with family and peers, so they have less experience with how to handle themselves in social situations. They've spent more time investing in the value of winning and less in the value of cooperating. They're lacking the very things that spending time with family would have provided for them.

The world of commerce is well aware that American parents are worried that they're not spending enough "family time" with their kids. Many theme parks have built advertising campaigns around the high-quality family time you'll have if you bring your kids for a visit. But who needs a world full of expensive fakery in order to have fun with family?

In a highly commoditized world, we've even come to see fun as a thing that you have to buy. But we could also teach our kids that fun is something you can make at home, even out of the simplest everyday tasks: growing a garden and cooking a meal. Unlike the expensive visit to the theme park, these activities yield something of benefit for the rest of the family.

Connections are forged, not just in expensive, highly artificial moments of contrived fun, but also in work shared. In striving together to get a meal on the table, kids learn about time management, problem solving, critical thinking, and division of labor. They develop the skills that are necessary to life in a group.

There's nothing wrong with buying a little fun now and then, but an exchange of money for entertainment can never enrich the soul the way an exchange of laughter, conversation, and ideas can. Buying fun tends to create dependency. *Making* fun creates self-reliance.

Local Food Strengthens Local Economies

What the local food lifestyle does for families, it also does for communities. When you buy your food from a supermarket, you engage in a short, sterile transaction with a stranger. You experience no connection to any part of the processes or people involved in bringing that food to you. Plus, the majority of every food dollar flows directly out of your community to enrich the coffers of a business that could be headquartered thousands of miles away.

In contrast, when you buy from a farmer or local business, you're interacting with a neighbor. There's a warmth in these transactions that goes beyond a sterile exchange at the cash register. When you invest your food budget in local businesses, the people who actually did the work get to hang on to a larger proportion of each dollar, and when they spend their share, they'll put a good chunk of it right back into the community.

For these reasons, local food fosters community cohesion in a way that industrial foods never could.

Food Security Is a Community Affair

On New Year's Eve of the very first year we met, my friend Meredith showed up on my doorstep and presented me with a surprise gift, all done up in Christmas wrapping. I unwrapped it to find a can of pitted prunes with a quarter taped to the top. She explained, "It's a German tradition: food and money in the coming year if ever you're in need. It's a way of saying I've got your back."

The ritual she brought me into is a gesture of friendship. What's going on here is caretaking, not commerce. The reciprocity that characterized human interactions before the rise of the market economy was based on relationships. It didn't work with strangers, only with people to whom you had connections.

One of the common criticisms of the dominant economic system we have today is that most economic exchanges are impersonal and remote. When I buy a box of cereal from the supermarket, I have zero connection to the farmers who grew the grains, the company that manufactured the product, the store that stocked it, or even the cashier who sold it to me. It's easy to have maximizing profit as your goal, so long as the people you're extracting profit from remain strangers. But if the people you do business with are your friends and neighbors, you're invested in their well-being.

Business with the primary goal of caretaking will probably never make anyone stinkin' rich, but it *can* make you an abundant living, at the same time that it strengthens bonds within your community.

Family Dinners Make for Happier, Healthier Kids

Many researchers are now confirming what Mom knew all along: kids who sit down at the dinner table with family most nights are reaping far greater benefits than just a nutritious meal. A 2012 study by University of Illinois professor Barbara Fiese, published in the journal *Economics and Human Biology*, shows that kids who ate meals at the family dinner table were less likely to be obese than those who ate in front of the TV, because at the table they were more likely to recognize the signs of fullness. By serving themselves from the dishes on the table, they also learned about portion size. Other recent studies have indicated that family dinners improve everything from children's social skills, vocabulary, and cognitive function to overall health and well-being, and make them less likely to smoke or use drugs.

It's for these reasons that, when we talk about food security and food self-sufficiency, it's a good idea to think on the scale of neighborhoods, towns, and communities, rather than on the scale of nations and regions. It needs to be addressed on a scale in which people know each other or, at least, feel that they have a responsibility to one another.

It may seem a little silly to be talking about food security here in the overfed United States, the wealthiest nation in the modern world. But food security is not just an issue of whether you can afford to eat, but also of who is doing the feeding. CEOs of major food corporations, who might never ingest the company's products or feed them to their own kids, certainly don't mind persuading you to feed the products to yours. They can make an outsized profit off providing you with nutritionally bankrupt food because they don't know you. They never have to look you in the eye. They'll never need to knock on your door at 6:00 a.m. for a battery jump. They've never sipped coffee with you at a PTA meeting.

In contrast, when the people you're feeding are your friends and neighbors, you're held accountable. You'll go the extra mile to ensure that the food you provide for them is as safe and nutritious as possible. You might slip an extra few potatoes into their sack because you remember the good turn they did for you last winter, or because you know their mother is ailing, or just because it really means something to you to keep their business.

When we talk about food security, we usually end up discussing logistical issues such as safety, distribution, and sustainability. But maybe it's just as important, in terms of social cohesion, that the people in a community are fed by someone who genuinely cares about their well-being.

A Future in Local Food: What Food-Based Connections Might Look Like Later in the Century

Just because we're talking about a shift to local food, I don't want you to think that means a return to the lifestyles of yesteryear. We've moved on from that cultural mind-set, so it would no longer be a fit with who we are. We'll really need to invent a new kind of local food culture, one that fits who we are today. I don't see this change in terms of cutting back, making do with less, or tightening our belts. I see it as a long conga line of new opportunities.

New Part-Time Community-Based Job Opportunities

According to investment manager and futurist James H. Lee, such a scenario will fit nicely with the working world as it's currently evolving. In his article "Hard at Work in a Jobless Future" in *Futurist* magazine, Lee predicts that, as the century progresses, we may see fewer people holding a single high-paying job. It may become the norm to work several part-time jobs with flexible hours and no fixed location. If Lee's picture of the future is correct, I can imagine an economic system in which one of the jobs in each person's portfolio might be *food-based*. In this case, local food fits quite nicely with the community of the future.

If Americans developed a new food culture dependent on small, local sources, many more people would have an opportunity to go into the food business. We'd need far more local farmers, butchers, bakers, and foodmakers of many kinds, plying their goods in the midst of their communities. This scenario presents a cornucopia of possibilities: rewarding work, lucrative income, and family-centric businesses.

Working families still need quick, cheap, healthy, portable lunches. A generation ago, a stay-at-home mom would have gotten up at 6:00 a.m. to pack the little brown bags for Dad and the kids. Today, many kids go to school with highly processed, highly packaged, and nutritionally bereft convenience lunches. Or just as bad, they may have to buy their lunches from the school cafeteria. But how about this alternative? On school days, in any given neighborhood, four parents seeking a little extra income meet at someone's house a couple of hours before bus time, whip up four hundred brown-bag lunches,—each with, for instance, a peanut butter and jelly sandwich, an apple, and some carrot sticks—and hand them out at neighborhood bus stops? They could collect a monthly fee from parents for this service. They could call it a school lunch co-op.

There might also be many more opportunities for kids to own and operate small business ventures: selling backyard produce or delivering it. Retired people, at-home parents, writers, teachers, and anyone else who is opting out of a traditional nine-to-five career would have an opportunity for simple, rewarding side work in providing food to their neighborhoods.

Food-Based Businesses Fit the 'Generative Economy'

Local food also fits in nicely with a rising trend in our economic system. Economist Marjorie Kelly coined the term "generative economy" to describe a national trend toward community-centric small businesses. In her book *Owning Our Future: The Emerging Ownership Revolution*, Kelly explains that what she terms "industrial-age capitalism" is causing financial and ecological turmoil, but at the same time, a new economic system is emerging, one that "serves the many rather than the few" and is "ecologically beneficial rather than harmful."

Kelly says the generative economy is already here and thriving, if only yet in its infancy. Its goal, she claims, "is not designed for the extraction of maximum financial wealth," but to "create the conditions for life." She compares generative business ownership, whose goal is to produce a modest but equitable and ecologically sustainable abundance, with our dominant system— the debt-driven business model she terms "extractive ownership," whose goal is to extract maximum financial wealth from the economy.

The generative economy Kelly envisions is driven by employee-owned businesses, cooperatives, and social enterprises, whose goals are to responsibly serve their communities. Local food, and the small, community-centric businesses it inspires, fit the generative economy perfectly.

If a generative economy is the wave of the future, then local food belongs to an economic model whose time has come.

Fried Fingers

My husband, Al, told me a story about the day his family got their first color TV, when they were living on Nagle Avenue in New York City. The neighbors mobbed their apartment, straining to get a look at the miraculous new device. He remembers this moment, less because of the TV, but because after everyone finally went home, his mom fixed one of his favorite childhood treats.

2 cups cornmeal

3 eggs

1 cup water

4 ounces grated Parmesan cheese

olive oil

Combine the cornmeal, eggs, cheese, and water. In a saucepan, boil the cornmeal mixture until you have a paste the consistency of clay. Divide the mix into golf-ball-sized globs and roll each into a finger shape. Fry each finger in olive oil, turning to brown both sides.

14

Closing the Loops

A Local Food Lifestyle Makes More Efficient Use of Natural Resources

The frog does not drink up the pond in which he lives. —*Native American Proverb*

In 2012, photographer David Liittschwager built a one-foot cube out of bright green metal tubing, placed it in various ecosystems around the world, and then photographed every living thing he found inside it for a twenty-four-hour period. He published his findings in his book *A World in One Cubic Foot: Portraits of Biodiversity*. His photographs give visual testimony to the astounding biodiversity on planet Earth. Everywhere he placed the cube—the Temae Reef, a Costa Rican rain forest, even in Central Park in New York City—he was able to capture hundreds of life forms. Everywhere, that is, except in a cornfield in Iowa where crops were produced through industrial agriculture. In this cube, he found *just five* life forms.

In the past seventy years, human activity has caused the extinction of thousands of species. At this point, species extinctions are outpacing species discoveries. We are losing more species than we are finding.

Extinction itself is nothing new. According to geologists, biologists, and paleontologists, Earth has gone through numerous mass extinctions throughout its history, caused by meteor strikes, supervolcanoes, and other factors. But this current event, which paleoanthropologist Richard Leakey labeled "The Sixth Extinction," is the first wave of mass extinction caused by a species. Never in the history of Earth has a single life form had such a profound effect on biosphere, atmosphere, landscape, or climate.

In the year 2000, atmospheric chemist Paul Crutzen proposed the idea that the proper name for the current geological era of Earth was the "Anthropocene," a term originally coined by ecologist Eugene F. Stoermer, because we humans are now the greatest influence on Earth's climate and ecosystems. Crutzen claimed that the Anthropocene began with the Industrial Revolution in the late eighteenth century, although some people who advocate the use of this term push it all the way back to the advent of agriculture, the first time in our history when human beings began making a significant impact on their environments.

During the Anthropocene era, the greenhouse gases we have released into the atmosphere by burning fossil fuels have triggered a global rise in temperatures. We're already seeing a rise in sea levels and a resulting shift in global weather patterns. If this trend continues to the point at which global temperatures rise by more than four degrees Celsius, we're looking at the potential collapse of many ecosystems across the globe. When can we expect this change? Laura B. Huhn and William Halal reported in *Futurist* magazine that, according to the data analysis organization TechCast, unless we alter our present course of activities the four-degree rise in temperature will most likely happen between the years 2050 and 2100. Our children and grandchildren will see it.

Our impact is this great because at no time in our history have we consumed as much as we do today. We live in a society in which it's considered normal to drive five miles to the gym to walk a mile on a treadmill. We throw away our kitchen scraps and then spend eight dollars on a bag of compost for the garden. We make drink containers out of materials that last for hundreds of years, use them for five minutes, and discard them. Our society has become a system of open loops. The result is that we are wasting an enormous amount of energy and precious resources.

The way that we modern-day Westerners consume resources and generate waste is not in sync with the way nature does things. In the natural world, every ecosystem creates a series of closed loops. Plants convert sunlight into energy and absorb nutrients through their roots, herbivores eat plants, carnivores eat herbivores, both plants and animals die and decompose, and then microorganisms and fungi break down their organic material so that it can go around the cycle again. Nothing is wasted. In nature, there is no such thing as trash.

In this chapter, I'll talk about a few farming techniques that work with the way nature does things, so that you can be on the lookout for local food producers who practice them. I'll also call out a couple of lifestyle choices that allow us to close a few of our own dangling environmental loops.

Last of the Wild

In 2002, the Wildlife Conservation Agency and the Center for International Earth Science Information Network estimated that the total amount of Earth's surface that is directly affected by human activity is 83 percent. Only 17 percent of Earth remains unaffected by humans, the very last of the wild.

It wouldn't be spot-on to assume that, just because we eat local, compost our kitchen scraps, and grow a mess of vegetables in the backyard each summer, we've achieved zero-environmental-impact, but these are some of the choices that move us toward a more sustainable lifestyle.

Does Technology Overcome the Need for Sustainability?

For the purposes of this discussion, we can say that sustainable farming is a way of producing food that doesn't deplete natural resources faster than nature can renew them, that doesn't substantively harm the land or the life forms in its environment, that allows the people who produce the food to make a decent living at it, and that adequately meets the caloric and nutritional needs of its community.

Sustainable food production sounds good, but it's a bit hard to achieve, particularly in a society that believes it needs to keep its economy growing. The general agreement among experts who study sustainability is that you can't have infinite economic growth when you live on a planet with finite resources.

Some experts have claimed that we can get around this roadblock because, as economies grow, technology innovations allow resources to be used more efficiently. There's certainly a degree of truth in this, and it has already happened many times. But it doesn't really solve the problem, because there's no guarantee that innovation is going to keep pace with the demands we place on natural resources, that an innovation is always going to show up just when it's needed and be disseminated everywhere it's needed, or that innovations can infinitely stretch finite resources.

In the end, we still need to live within our means. No amount of technological innovation gives us enough escape velocity to completely get away from the need for a sustainable way of life.

Industrial Agriculture: A System of Broken Loops

The hallmark of industrial agriculture is its dependence on artificial inputs: resources that can't be produced on site, but which must be manufactured, purchased, and brought in from outside the farm.

Industrial agriculture is made possible only by an abundance of cheap fossil fuels. Petroleum runs the machinery necessary to till, plant, and harvest massive tracts of farmland. It drives the transportation that carries its produce to market, hundreds or thousands of miles from where it was grown.

According to the United Nation's Food and Agriculture Organization (FAO), agriculture accounts for 30 percent of energy use worldwide. Without these artificial inputs, this massive system of food production would be impossible. Undeniably, this system produces an enormous amount of food. But when the advocates of industrial agriculture sing its praises, they seldom factor in its true environmental cost.

Industrial agriculture depletes natural resources at a faster rate than nature can replenish them. Geographer-biologist Jared Diamond, in his book *Collapse: How Societies Choose to Fail or Succeed*, calls this procedure "mining." We usually use this word to refer to the extraction of minerals, but Diamond argues that it can be applied to any system that leaves its environment at a deficit. By Diamond's definition, industrial agriculture counts as a form of mining, because it extracts fossil fuels, soil fertility, and biodiversity at a nonrenewable rate.

Industrial agriculture is also notorious for polluting soil, air, and water. Obviously, the burning of fossil fuels that run the machinery of industrial agriculture releases carbon dioxide into the air, but industrial agriculture pollutes its environment in other ways as well. Excess artificial fertilizer runs off and ends up in streams and lakes, where it fertilizes algae blooms that deplete oxygen and kill fish. The pesticides, fungicides, and herbicides that industrial farmers spray on to their crops don't vanish after spraying, but also make their way into water and soil.

The threat of harm from industrial agriculture is not just an abstract prediction about a bleak future. It's happening *now*. According to the FAO, 25 percent of the world's farmland has already suffered loss of productivity as a result of unsustainable practices. This has led to desertification, erosion, loss of soil fertility, and salinization.

By our definition of sustainability, there's no question that, at least for now, industrial agriculture produces enough calories to meet the nutritional requirements of our nation. But by all other parts of the definition—conservation of resources, minimal impact to ecosystems, and economic benefits to its laborers—it fails miserably.

For comparison, let's look at a few of the farming techniques that ecologically minded small farmers favor.

Backyard Beekeepers Wanted!

Over the past decade, the world has seen a mass die-off of European honeybees, *apis mellifera*, the primary species farmers rely on for crop pollination. The phenomenon has a name: colony collapse disorder. Although speculations abound, no one is sure what's causing it yet. But it has been decimating 30 percent to 90 percent of bee colonies annually since 2007.

Until we work out a cure for what's ailing the bees, backyard beekeeping enthusiasts are in high demand. Their smaller, isolated apiaries may help to contain the disease. If you join the ranks of amateur beekeepers, you could help preserve the world's honeybees, enjoy higher pollination rates in your garden, and savor some of the finest honey on the planet. For information about beekeeping, visit the Backyard Beekeepers Association at www.beeculture.com.

Small-Scale Farming Leaves a Lighter Footprint

The USDA defines the size of farms not by acreage but by revenue, with a "small" farm being one that brings in less than $250,000 a year. By this definition, more than 90 percent of American farms are small. But perhaps more useful for our purposes is the physical size of the farm. Although there doesn't seem to be an official size, most definitions I found consider a small farm to be ten acres or smaller.

Advocates of industrial farming argue that small-scale farming simply isn't practical from an economic standpoint, because it couldn't possibly be as profitable as a large-scale operation. Yet, some evidence suggests that small farms may actually be more lucrative than large ones. Global food and farming activist Peter M. Rosset argued this point by referencing a U.S. Agricultural Census from 1992 that compared the average net profit per acre per season of different-sized farms. The net per acre was highest for the smallest farms and declined steadily as the number of acres rose. A farm of less than four acres saw an average net of $1,400 per acre, while a farm of 6,709 acres averaged only $12 per acre.

Organic Farming Uses Natural Inputs

The label "organic gardener" once prompted the laying-on of other labels, such as "hippie," "tree hugger," and similar terms that were less-than-respectfully meant. Today, with generations of quiet success behind them, organic gardeners are now almost as likely to wear labels such as "smart" and "forward-thinking."

Whenever possible, organic farmers avoid introducing artificial inputs to their food-growing environments. They don't burn the soil with chemical fertilizers. They abstain from chemical pesticides and herbicides because of their toxicity. They don't feed their livestock hormones or routine antibiotics. Instead, they try to accomplish soil fertility, pest control, and animal health with natural inputs they can produce on-site.

Many organic gardeners try to leave the soil as undisturbed as possible, so that it can develop its own natural integrity and complexity. Instead of tilling, they prefer to add regular top-dressings of compost and mulch, and then let earthworms drag this rich organic matter deep down into the soil. Organic gardeners prefer to rely on their own composted garden scraps, kitchen waste, and animal manure to add fertility to their soils.

Organic gardeners don't automatically view weeds and bugs as pests. Some weeds may help control erosion and preserve moisture, and some beneficial bugs may help control the ones that are pests. Instead of treating their plants with artificial chemicals, they interplant compatible species and rotate crops to stay one step ahead of pests and pathogens. They sometimes whip up their own homemade pest deterrents concocted from hot chilies, soap, garlic, and teas brewed from plants that insect pests find nasty.

The mind-set of an organic gardener is that healthy plants and animals are naturally disease resistant. They tend to believe that it's smarter to work *with* Mother Nature, rather than against her.

A growing number of U.S. farms have achieved the USDA Organic certification, but because this process is painstaking and exacting, and takes a minimum of three years, you'll often find farms that are unofficially organic. They don't have the official certification, but they try to be as organic in their practices as they possibly can.

Diversified Farming Stands Strong Against Adversity

Where the industrial agriculture system favors monoculturing—the large-scale growing of a single crop—small-scale growers are more likely to choose diversified farming, raising many different kinds of fruits, vegetables, and animals in a mutually beneficial system. One of the drawbacks of monoculture is that if any given season brings conditions that cause the crop to fail, the impact is enormous. "Diversity gets you through the good years and the bad," organic farmer Nick Maravell explains. His farm grows a range of crops and animals. Some tolerate drought, while others can handle a chilly, wet season. "We like diversity in our customer base, too," Nick says. "Everything fits everything else."

Where the industrial system tends to concentrate on producing the highest possible yields, small, diversified farms are managed for the highest yield the land can sustain. To illustrate this difference, Nick draws a distinction between *maximizing* and *optimizing*: "Maximizing deals only with one component of a farm at a time. It masks nature's systemic response. Optimizing seeks stability by emphasizing naturally occurring and self-regulating system dynamics." He agrees that high yields are important, but he notes that they have to be placed in the context of overall system health.

Grass Farming Builds Vibrant Soil

The livestock-raising technique known as grass farming mimics the natural cycles found on Earth's savannas. On the prairie, herds of herbivores, as they're migrating and being chased around by predators, stimulate regrowth with their grazing, aerate the soil with their trampling hooves, and fertilize the area with their nutrient-rich dung. Flocks of birds follow behind the herds, providing pest control by eating the larvae from the dung. The grass farmer simulates these conditions by moving the herds frequently and bringing chickens or turkeys along behind them. This method creates vigorous topsoil and grass with deep, healthy roots that green up faster in the spring, remain green longer into the winter, and are highly resistant to drought. Grass farming can rebuild depleted soils and heal erosion. With this method, an area too fragile to support tillage may still produce pastured milk, meat, and eggs while its topsoil recovers.

Permaculture Farming Takes Its Cues From Natural Cycles

The farming technique known as permaculture was developed in the 1970s by Australians Bill Mollison and David Holmgren, and it is practiced around the globe today. Permaculture techniques are modeled after natural ecosystems. They operate with a minimum of external inputs and human labor. Permaculture farms "harvest" rainwater in barrels, ponds, and swales for irrigation, and they emphasize the planting of perennials rather than annual crops that need to be resown into tilled soil each year.

These farms grow a variety of items together at the same time. They grow diversified crops in multiple layers and make use of vertical as well as horizontal spaces. Permaculture gardens look like crowded riots of growing things, and hence are often described as "food forests."

Permaculture farming isn't just a collection of nature-inspired growing techniques. It's also an ethic, one that connects farmers and their neighbors. These folks help each other out with farm tasks, exchange seeds in "seed libraries," build community food forests, share food in "crop swaps," and donate their surplus produce to local food banks. Many permaculture farms offer CSAs (community supported agriculture programs) to their communities.

So, What Do These Farming Methods Have to Do With Eating Local Food?

Food you buy directly from a small-scale grower is far more likely to have been produced by one or more of the methods we've just discussed. Because they're local, you can visit the farm site and see for yourself that their techniques are environmentally sound. By buying your food from these local small-scale producers, you're automatically lightening your family's environmental footprint.

How to Close a Few More Loops

The fastest route to a lower-impact way of eating is to start buying as much of your food as you can from local, sustainable sources. To make your environmental footprint even lighter, here are a few other things you can do:

Buy Whole, Unpackaged, and Delivered. Save on gas and avoid the temptation to buy non-local stuff by having your local food delivered. Whenever possible, avoid packaging by buying your food in a whole, natural state. Do your own cooking and combining of ingredients.

Grow 25 Percent of What Your Family Consumes. Use whatever sunny space you have available and set yourself the task of producing about one-fourth of your family's fresh fruit and vegetables during the growing season. Even if all you have is a wall or a windowsill, you can take advantage of urban gardening and permaculture techniques. It's amazing how much you can grow in a small amount of space.

Compost Your Kitchen Scraps and Yard Waste. With scrap lumber, build a three-bay compost bin about three feet high, open at the front. Into the first bay, toss kitchen scraps and yard waste, everything except animal products. Layer "greens" (plant scraps) with "browns" (dried grass, cardboard, and mulch). When that one is full, let it "cook" while you fill up the next bay. By the time you fill the third one, the first pile will probably be ready to go onto your garden. You'll know it's ready when it stops looking and smelling like kitchen trash and resembles rich, peaty soil. If you live in an apartment, or you just don't like the idea of handling smelly, drippy, decomposing food,

Is It Safe?

We import 50 percent of fruits and 20 percent of vegetables from abroad. Only 2 percent of imported fruits and vegetables are inspected.

A Call for Environmental Enlightenment

The average American, myself included, is astonishingly uninformed about our effect on the natural world. We're disconnected from the sources of the products we buy, the processes by which they're manufactured, the means by which they travel to us, and the fate of these same materials once we discard them. We tend to rely on messages from the corporate world for information about the environmental impact of the products we buy. Unfortunately, this is not an impartial source.

Daniel Goleman, author of *Ecological Intelligence*, writes that it's difficult for us to see that the items we buy and use each day "have other kinds of costs," namely, their costs to the planet. He warns of the danger of thinking that just because we recycle a few plastic bags, we're living green. It's not that simple.

If we're going to find a way for several billion humans to live equitably and sustainably on this planet, we'll need to take people's environmental awareness as seriously as we take their education in any other subject. Because of the technological power we now wield, we cannot afford to be ignorant of our effect on the planet.

From now on, we'll need to insist that manufacturers and retailers fully inform us about the impact their products have on the environment. Economist Joseph Stiglitz claims that consumer ignorance damages the efficiency of the market, and that a truly healthy economic system runs on an accurate exchange between seller and consumer.

This disclosure of information, which Goleman calls "radical transparency," is needed in all the products that we buy, but it's especially important when it comes to food. You could hardly name another item that has such a profound impact on so many aspects of human life, from health, safety, nutrition, and well-being to community cohesion, economic stability, environmental conservation, and sustainability.

---

there's a new trend afoot that might serve you well: urban compost pickup services. For a fee, these folks will collect your organic non-meat kitchen waste, typically in a bin you leave outside your door. With certain caveats, they may also deliver a share of the finished compost for your gardening needs—though you can opt out of this part of the deal if you don't garden. To find a service near you, search "compost pickup service" on the Internet.

Save Your Seeds. Let one or two of your best-producing plants go to seed and harvest them for next year. Scoop seeds out of fruits. Rinse them and lay them out in a pie pan to dry for a few weeks, then label and bag them for next year's garden.

Let Your Chickens Do the Fertilizing and Pest Control. A backyard flock of chickens will eat your kitchen scraps, reduce the bug population, and fertilize your topsoil, all while providing you with plenty of fresh, tasty eggs. To find out whether you can have chickens where you live, call your local economic development office.

100 Percent or Nothing?

I've read criticisms of various farming techniques that denounce them for not being 100 percent sustainable. But how can we truly know for certain whether *any* form of food production is completely sustainable? Rather than thinking in terms of all or nothing, could we think instead of sustainability as a process? Could we think of learning, choosing, and changing over time?

We're looking at a difference between what it would be ideal to do and what, realistically, it's *possible* to do. It's unknown whether several billion human beings can live sustainably on Earth. But it's an absolute certainty that we can live more sustainably than we have been.

Virginia Peanut Cookies

Did you know you can grow peanuts in your backyard? We did, just last summer. They'll grow almost anywhere, north to south, as long as they're planted in full sunlight after the last frost. Just like peas and beans, they put nitrogen in the soil, so your garden will love them. Plus, homegrown, fresh-roasted peanuts beat anything you can buy from the store. I adapted my son Ben's peanut butter cookie recipe to showcase these marvelous little ground-dwelling nuggets.

1 cup Virginia peanuts, shelled and roasted

1 cup flour

3/4 cup honey

1/4 cup oil

1 egg

1 tablespoon vanilla extract

1/2 teaspoon baking soda

1/4 teaspoon nutmeg

1/4 teaspoon salt

Blend the honey together with the egg and vanilla extract. In a separate bowl, combine the flour, baking soda, nutmeg and salt. Gradually combine the dry ingredients with the egg mixture. Add the peanuts and stir. Drop spoonfuls of the batter onto a greased baking sheet. Bake at 375 degrees until lightly brown, usually less than ten minutes.

15

Dinner for Ten Billion

How Local Food Supports an Equitable World Economy

The class of citizen who provide at once their own food and their own raiment may be viewed as the most truly independent and happy. —*James Madison*

This past semester, one of my anthropology students had this to say in a social issues paper: "I went to a diner once and ordered some toast. I asked the waitress if they had marmalade. She brought me the one last packet of marmalade they had. It wasn't much. I had to ask myself, do I spread it so thin that each bite has very little flavor, or just cut the toast in half, enjoying one particularly tasty side, while leaving the other dry and bland? I think of our planetary resources like that little packet of marmalade, and the toast like the world population. In the end, you can only spread the marmalade so thin over the toast, and there just ain't enough to go around."

By sheer numbers, the picture does indeed look bleak. According to the United Nations' Food and Agriculture Organization, in a world of more than seven billion people, nearly 870 million suffer chronic undernourishment. According to the United Nations, the world's population will continue to grow, by quite a bit, before the growth trend levels off. By 2050, Earth may be home to as many as 10.6 billion of us. How will we feed them all, if we're not adequately feeding everyone who is around today?

The student who wrote that paper was envisioning a world in which some of us have all the "marmalade" we want, while others don't have the means to get enough. Yet, who among us would voluntarily resort to spreading our own too thin, just so others can have a little more?

Because we're cut off from experiencing the true effects of our consumption, we Westerners have become accustomed to consuming as much of any given resource as we want. That ride appears to be coming to an end.

According to futurist Michael Klare, certain resources that have always been abundant are now beginning to run short. In his book *Race for What's Left,* he notes that we're already seeing competition for water, oil, farmland, and minerals. Why are we running out of these things? Simply because, as Klare puts it, although "populations and economies can grow exponentially, the planet's resources cannot."

According to Klare, a few nations are already competing for arable land: China, India, South Korea, and Saudi Arabia and other Persian Gulf countries are buying foreign farmland to produce food for their own people. Most of the land they're buying is in sub-Saharan Africa, and much of it is already in use by pastoralists and hunter-gatherers, who will likely be forced off the land and into poverty.

It surely looks like we're coming to the end of easy access to oil, too. Journalist Nafeez Ahmed reported in a 2013 article for the *Guardian* that, according to retired BP geologist Dr. Richard G. Miller, the world's reserves of conventional oil probably *already* peaked in 2008. New oil harvesting techniques, such as deep water drilling and tar sands extraction, are now tapping fresh sources of oil, but these require more intensive extraction methods. And if we do pull all that unconventional oil out of the ground and burn it, climate scientists say the result will be catastrophic climate change.

A similar story is playing out with the world's access to freshwater. According to the World Health Organization and UNICEF, approximately 780 million people worldwide don't have access to clean drinking water. The Ogallala Aquifer in North America, which provides water for much of the Midwest's grain production, is beginning to show signs of depletion in certain places. This underground water source was deposited by glacial melt from the last ice age, and once it's gone, it won't be coming back.

Although the 21st century has yet to see massive global food shortages or catastrophic crop failures, there's some evidence to suggest we're beginning to tap out the fertility of the soil we depend on for crop production. According to the FAO, 25 percent of the world's farmland has already suffered loss of productivity because of overtilling and other unsustainable practices.

So, what's going on here? Why are we beginning to run short of the resources we've always enjoyed in abundance? When I pose this question to my students, the answer I get back most frequently is "too many humans."

Are they right?

Have We Maxed Out Earth's Carrying Capacity for Humans?

Could it be that Earth simply has more humans than it can sustain? The more people there are on the planet, the more acute the problems of providing for us all. Many anthropologists assert that Earth has already reached its carrying capacity for humans. In ecological terms, "carrying capacity" refers to the maximum population of a species that *a given environment* can support. But in this case, we're talking about the total capacity of the *planet*. Scientists who think we're already at carrying capacity point to the fact that there are already many people around the world today who starve.

I'm not sure I agree. There's far more to this equation than simply the number of humans on the planet compared with the amount of food. Human lifestyles vary *enormously* from one place to the next. Some ways of living make a much greater impact on their environments than others. National Geographic's Human Footprint project claims that if everyone lived as we Westerners do, we would need more than four additional Earths to keep up with the demand on resources. By contrast, if all human beings lived in the manner of the average modern Bangladeshi, the Earth's total carrying capacity for humans would be much higher.

In fact, the parts of the world that are expecting the most growth in population within coming decades are those in which the current lifestyle is lower-impact than ours. It's certainly not because all those folks are choosing to live a green lifestyle. In most cases, they're consuming less because they don't have the economic means to consume more.

The precise number of humans Earth can handle is not a matter of one simple equation. We also need to consider how those human beings make their living. Making a lower impact doesn't necessarily demand a monastic lifestyle, but it does require us to make conscious and well-informed consumption choices.

But If Earth Can Feed Us All, Why Does Anyone Go Hungry?

As I come to understand more about the economic history of the twentieth century, I can see that, in many cases, people *did* starve as a result of a sheer lack of food in their region. For instance, in the 1950s and the

Does Mr. Malthus Deserve Such a Bad Rap?

In 1798, economist Thomas Malthus predicted the inevitable demise of humankind because, to boil it down, human populations can expand practically without limit, yet we've never figured out how to grow more farmland. Malthus has been strongly denounced because his theory failed to account for human innovation, which has massively increased the productive capacity of farmland. We can get far more out of an acre today than we could in Malthus's day.

If you were to suggest that seven billion humans might be stretching Earth's carrying capacity, somebody might just call you a "Malthusian," and they probably don't mean it as a compliment.

But could Mr. Malthus have been partly right? Is there any law, natural or economic, that assures that an agricultural innovation will show up just when we need it, that it will provide the required amount of expansion in food supply, that the benefits of the innovation will be applied equitably, or that the innovation that saves us in the short run will not prove damaging to the environment in the long run?

decades that followed it, human populations rose so quickly that world food production struggled to keep up. But there's another dynamic at play here that explains why, even in the face of abundant food resources, people can still go hungry.

Today, in many parts of the world where people aren't getting enough to eat, it's often because they don't have equitable access to resources. You can't buy land, tools, and seeds without money. You can't earn money without a job. These places lack the social, political, and economic structures that enable people to purchase or produce their own food. They're not facing a shortage of *food*, but a shortage of *equality*. In these cases, ample food may be present in the area, but if you're one of the people living there, the question of whether or not you have access to it depends on who you are. Although famines may begin because of a drought or population pressure, the political factor is equally important: food may be withheld from a population because of war, oppression, or governmental mismanagement.

In many cases, the reasons any group struggles to feed itself are rooted in history. For instance, in *Food First: Beyond the Myth of Scarcity*, authors Frances Moore Lappé and Joseph Collins explain that, in recent centuries, colonial governments forcibly turned subsistence farms into cash-crop plantations. Many colonized people, who were previously able to feed themselves from their own lands, were then removed to marginal areas or forced to sell their labor cheaply.

The inherent flaw in any scenario that forces people to meet their needs by selling their labor is that there's nothing to guarantee that there will be enough jobs for everyone, or that those jobs will pay sufficient wages. Even today, the descendants of the people affected by colonial domination often lack access to sufficient economic resources.

Wherever we find hungry people, a simple handout of food is not enough, because "lack of food" is not the whole story. We need to understand the real reasons why any given group of people is unable to own sufficient land, equipment, resources, and financial capital to feed itself. If a group is facing a crisis, we may need to assist them with food donations in the short run. But our ultimate goal is to remove the barriers to food self-sufficiency.

How Do We Prepare to Feed Ten Billion?

Global competition for resources, environmental crises, inequality—do we have reasons to be pessimistic? Maybe. But we also have choices.

When I first started studying anthropology, one of the very first questions I asked was, "Are human beings getting *better?* Is our species improving over time?" Of course, it's hard to respond to a question like that scientifically, because how do you define and measure a broad, subjective term such as "better"? But I've come to realize that when I try to understand human beings, I always make a certain assumption, a positive one, and it turns out there's actually a word for it.

Meliorism, according to Webster's Dictionary, is "the assumption that the world is getting better over time, and that humans can aid its betterment." I've decided to be a meliorist. I'm taking it on faith that, even though humankind may be on the brink of many significant challenges, overall we're on the right track. Along the way, I've bumped into some compelling evidence to support this belief. For instance, Steven Pinker, in his book *The Better Angels of Our Nature*, makes the case that, in spite of some of the darker episodes of the recent human past, we're headed toward a future with less violence, more knowledge, more respect for human rights, more tolerance of differences, and a better quality of life. We're better equipped now to tackle problems on a global scale than we've ever been before.

So, given what we're up against, how do we assure that everyone is properly fed, today and in the future? As I've read more about this issue, I've come to believe that the best way for people to eat, whether in the Industrialized West or elsewhere, is to have both access to a global food system and the opportunity to get as much of their own food as possible from small, local producers—in fact, to produce as much of their own food as possible, wherever it's practical. Global food access safeguards against regional calamity; local food access solves the distribution problem, strengthens communities, and allows people to see and learn for themselves how their food was raised.

As a card-carrying meliorist, I'm taking it on faith that it *is* possible to feed ten billion people and more, locally and sustainably, but to do this we will have to rethink our notion of efficiency: what's expedient for the short term may not be what's most efficient for the long term. The plan that generates the maximum profit may not be the same as the one that feeds everyone regardless of their ability to pay.

Does Wealth Equal Well-being?

The well-being of a society is not merely a matter of gross domestic product or average per capita income, but of how securely, equitably, sustainably, and abundantly the needs of its people are met. Economic abundance in a given society has enormous potential to aid well-being, but it can only do so to the extent that its members have equitable access to it.

Instead of thinking "biggest, fastest, and most profitable," we've got to redefine "efficiency" as "safely provides abundant nutrition, feeds everyone equitably, and doesn't use up tomorrow's resources to produce today's food."

The best way to grow food sustainably is to do it on a small, local scale, with diversified farming that relies on few outside inputs and takes its cues from natural cycles. And, to the extent that every community has the means to produce its own food close to home, with this system there are no worries about distribution.

This, then, is the ultimate goal: to support *community food security* by supplementing access to global food with local food production worldwide. How do we do this, and on what scale? When I think in terms of my own sphere of influence, I envision three concentric circles: local, national, and international. Or, put another way, my community, my country, and my planet. I try to focus my efforts on each of these levels. Here's how this looks:

Local Food for Hungry Neighbors: Feeding the Folks Around Home. I just have a very strong feeling that, even as I'm helping hungry people in faraway lands, I also want to be doing something to take care of the folks back home.

Even in a well-off state such as Maryland, there are places where people have a tough time feeding themselves. The USDA reports that more than 720,000 Marylanders aren't sure where their next meal is coming from. Thankfully, there's no shortage of local opportunities to get involved in feeding people. My area is blessed with a cornucopia of food banks, community-donated CSA shares, and many other organizations and programs that get food to people who need it. The Maryland Food Bank, a statewide affiliate of Feeding America, distributes 79,000 meals to hungry Marylanders every day. If you're looking to get involved in your community's food outreach organizations, search for them on the Internet by typing in the name of your town or county and the words "food bank."

Local Food for the United States: Spreading the Wealth of the Richest Nation. In the United States, arguably the richest nation on the planet, nobody starves to death, but according to the USDA, not everyone in the nation gets enough food to maintain optimum health. In 2011, 14.9 percent of American households experienced food insecurity at some point during the year, meaning that their eating patterns were disrupted because they didn't have enough money for food. If we're so prosperous, and food is so abundant, how is it that we're not even properly feeding all of our own?

Many of our nation's poorest citizens live in urban centers where access to fresh, whole food is limited. There are fast food restaurants and convenience shops in these neighborhoods, but it's impossible to find a fresh head of lettuce or a pound of broccoli. The residents of these neighborhoods often don't have cars, so they can't simply drive out to the nearest farmers' market.

Restoring food security to these "food deserts" is a work in progress. First Lady Michelle Obama has encouraged retailers to open shops in areas where fresh food is scarce, and as the success stories for this strategy accumulate, more grocery chains may be persuaded to follow suit. Some private businesses and city programs have brought in mobile food pantries—literally, farmers' markets on wheels—as well as food carts that sell fresh fruits and vegetables instead of hot dogs and fries. Online CSAs and buyers' clubs can arrange delivery to neighborhoods that are currently underserved. The urban gardening movement is flourishing in many inner cities, greening up

Why Do We Need Public Food Assistance in a Nation Where Even the Poor Are Obese?

In 2013, a great deal of Internet conversation sprung up around proposed cuts to the federal Supplemental Nutritional Assistance Program (SNAP). Many voices in the debate questioned why nutritional assistance was necessary at all in a nation that each day produces several hundred calories more per person than we need. They were quick to point out that some of the worst examples of the country's obesity epidemic could be found among the lowest income people in the nation. Why do we need to give food handouts, they reasoned, to people who are already so fat?

The reason obesity is a larger problem among the lowest income earners is that the cheapest and most readily available food in the nation is processed industrial food. The stuff that packs on the most pounds for the least amount of nutritional benefit is the only kind of food many people can afford on a day-to-day basis. Fresh produce is priced beyond the means of many lower-income Americans.

Among the urban poor, the problem is compounded by a lack of access to fresh food. Even the poorest neighborhoods are home to fast food restaurants and convenience stores on almost every block, but there's no place to buy fresh fruits and vegetables. This situation has given rise to the term "food desert" to describe an area where fresh, healthy food is difficult to find.

abandoned lots and rooftops and turning them into sources of fresh food as well as community meeting places.

If you're looking to get involved, you can volunteer with or donate to hunger relief organizations such as Oxfam America and Feeding America, which serve U.S. populations in need.

Local Food Across Nations: Fostering Food Security Abroad. In coming decades, the parts of the world that will need the most help feeding their people are those places that are already struggling with food insecurity, and whose youthful populations are poised to grow exponentially. These places include much of sub-Saharan Africa and Southeast Asia. We already know that growth is imminent in these places, so the time to get a plan in place is now.

When we hear that people are going hungry, our first impulse is to ship massive amounts of food aid to them. But although such a measure might arguably be necessary in the short run, food aid by itself does little to address the root cause of the problem, which comes down to people being shut out of access to the land, cash, tools, and other resources needed to reliably buy or grow their own food. If we want people to produce their own food securely, these are the problems we must tackle. In fact, blindly dumping food aid, without a plan for helping people break their reliance on it, may be more of a detriment than a help, because it discourages the development of local food economies.

On the international scene, many excellent charities focus not just on providing a handout but a hand *up*. They advocate for people's rights to farmable land. They provide communities with seeds, tools, livestock, and basic agrarian knowledge. Programs such as Save the Children, Heifer Project International, and Oxfam International bring resources for self-sufficiency into impoverished communities.

What Else Can We Do?

If you can afford to buy good local food yourself, by all means, please do. Ben Hewlett, in the book *The Town That Food Saved*, claims that local food may have to live with an "artisanal" stigma for the time being, because it can't compete with the mass production of industrial food. But the more of us who buy it, the cheaper and more abundant it will become.

To conserve resources while we're working our way through this temporary environmental bottleneck, many people advocate eating less meat.

Raising meat CAFO-style, by feeding the animals grains grown on land that could have grown food for humans, is inherently wasteful. But neither could we simply turn all those CAFO animals loose on open pasture and go on eating meat at our current consumption level. Every population of animals has a threshold of sustainability, which is determined by the environment it's raised in. Instead of eating all the meat we want, we'll need to learn to eat the amount of meat we can raise sustainably, whatever that turns out to be.

If we learn to live on less meat, that may not be such a bad thing. John Robbins, author of *The Food Revolution*, claims that vegetarians have fewer heart attacks; fewer instances of heart disease, high blood pressure, and diabetes; and are far less likely to be obese than habitual meat eaters. The statistics are even better for vegans, people who eat no animal products at all. I asked my family doctor if her experience confirmed this: were vegetarians really that much healthier than meat eaters? She responded enthusiastically in the affirmative and, as a vegetarian herself, passed along her recipe for butternut squash lasagna.

You may not have to go full-on vegan to benefit from better health. Even relegating meat to a smaller corner of your diet will improve the way you feel. Thomas Jefferson advocated using meat as a flavoring rather than a main course. Doing this just a couple nights a week will reduce your meat consumption without making you feel deprived.

We might also choose to help people, especially kids, reconnect with nature. Because of the scope of our impact on the natural world, we have a responsibility to educate ourselves about it. Ours is the first generation to be almost completely nature-illiterate, and we can't afford that. Richard Louv, in his book *The Nature Principle,* makes the case for a new medical syndrome that he calls "nature-deficit disorder." He claims there's a growing gap between children and nature that must be remedied. The more technological our lives become, the more exposure to nature we'll need in order to stay in balance.

Nature, Louv claims, makes fuller use of our faculties. It gives us a sense of humility and increases our intelligence. Time spent in nature also enhances physical and emotional health and family bonding. A 2008 study by Janice F. Bell, Jeffrey S. Wilson, and Gilbert C. Liu published in the *American Journal of Preventive Medicine* showed that kids who grew up in neighborhoods with green spaces averaged a lower body mass index score.

As an enrichment teacher, I'm fortunate to work with kids directly. I've been able to create classes and activities that get them outside, engaged with nature, and learning about living things and the way food grows. A few years back, I started "grading" their snacks—a D-minus for a pack of gummi candies, an A-plus for a bag of apple slices. It began as a joke, but after a while, I noticed the kids were bringing me their snacks for grading, and they seemed proud when a whole food they'd brought from home earned a good grade.

If you're looking for a chance to help kids engage with nature, there's no shortage of volunteer opportunities, anywhere in the United States, that will allow you to do just that. Scouting organizations, local schools, and youth groups of all kinds would be happy to have you as a volunteer.

Toward a Future Where All Are Fed

We're facing some hefty challenges in the near future. But the human species is nothing if not resilient. In our past, every time we've faced some new threat to our survival, we've risen to the task and invented a new way of life for ourselves.

Human history, when viewed through the longest possible lens, is a story of one remarkable innovation after another, each building on the one before. Two million years ago, our ancestors invented the hunter-gatherer lifestyle that enabled them to range across a vast variety of ecosystems, adapting their lifestyles as they went. Eleven thousand years ago, our forebears began to grow their own food, allowing for the building of permanent settlements. Five and a half thousand years ago, a new form of society—the state—enabled a synergy of knowledge and ideas that eventually gave rise to science and the arts. Five hundred years ago, the Enlightenment triggered a rise in empathy and human rights. A hundred years ago, petroleum power spurred the growth of modern industry and science. Fifty years ago, the communications revolution connected human beings on a global scale, and for the first time we were able to become a truly international society.

Today, we're on the threshold of another revolution in human history. We have a chance to achieve a new era in which the sovereign right of every person is respected, and everyone's basic needs are amply met. We have a chance, for the first time in our history, to act as a species. Instead of remaining a threat to our planet, we have the opportunity to become its guardians and champions. I believe we'll rise to the occasion.

100 Clove Garlic Soup

100 garlic cloves

3 cups onions, finely diced

8 cups chicken or vegetable stock

1 cup fresh cream

4 tablespoons butter

4 tablespoons olive oil

4 tablespoons fresh oregano

1 cup grated fresh Parmesan cheese

Put half of the garlic cloves—skin-on—in a casserole dish, sprinkle with olive oil and salt, and bake at 325 degrees for about 30 minutes or until lightly brown. Set aside and let cool.

Put the onions, oregano, and butter in a large pot and cook about five minutes on medium. Peel both the roasted and raw garlic cloves and place all of them in the pot. Cook on low heat for five more minutes. Pour in the stock, cover, and let cook on low heat for 30 minutes.

Let the soup cool a little, and then place it in a food processor or blender, on purée, for about a minute. Place the soup back in the pot. Add the cream. Warm the soup on a very low heat. Pour into bowls and add a sprinkling of Parmesan cheese to each bowl.

16

Defending Local Food

How to Respond to Your Critics

When you do things from your soul, you feel a river moving in you, a joy. —*Rumi*

When people find out you're eating differently than they do, that there's a distinctive worldview and an informed choice driving your food life, they'll have questions for you. Many will be impressed and want to know how you do it. A few—*just a few*—may argue, call you names, and try to verbally take you down for holding a point of view that is different from theirs.

I've devoted this last chapter to the voices that oppose local food, because making a truly informed choice also means understanding the objections to that choice. I'll be talking about some of the deeply held beliefs within our contemporary culture that tend to bias us against local food. I'll also touch on a few of the arguments you're likely to hear if you go through the world espousing a different way of eating, and some of the labels that people may try to hang on you as a result of your choice.

The Worldview You're Challenging

In contemporary America, big business has the ability to speak with a loud voice, and to weave its agenda into public policy. As a result, the corporate worldview has largely become the worldview of the average American citizen, perhaps, to an extent, without our even being aware of it. Our worldviews are often invisible to us, the way water is invisible to a fish. Even though we're immersed in our collective interpretations of reality, we're seldom conscious of them. That makes them a little bit difficult to examine and question. What follows are a few of the perspectives I've bumped into that appear to run contrary to the worldview inherent in local-sustainable food:

The American Dream Is About Being Able to Buy Whatever You Want.
At the heart of the American ethos is the notion that every citizen should have
the opportunity to achieve financial prosperity. That sounds like a great idea
to me. But if we put this value at the helm of a society that is rapidly commod-
itizing—placing a monetary value on an increasing number of the things that
people want and need—we produce a powerful drive to *spend* that wealth.
Add to this mix an advertising culture that relentlessly ties people's self-es-
teem to the stuff they buy—you've got to drive this car, wear that designer
label, live this high-consumption lifestyle to prove to the world that you're a
success—and what you get is a strong tendency to view high consumption
as the right of the prosperous.

   If, by my lifestyle, I seem to be advocating modest consumption, some
people may interpret this as an indictment of their own choice to consume
conspicuously. If consumption is the measure of success, to defer consumption might look like an invitation to failure, or at least, to *looking* like a failure,
and it's important for them to view themselves as a success, as they define it.

   Just to clarify, I'm not anti-consumption; I'm pro-conscientious-con-
sumption. I don't see this issue as a choice between asceticism and gluttony;
I'm hoping to make room for a third alternative. I'm aware of the need to
curb our consumption in the face of dwindling resources. But I keep thinking
there's got to be a way to live within the carrying capacity of our planet and
still enjoy abundance. I suspect it has mostly to do with the way we *define*
abundance.

Big Business Creates Wealth for the Whole Nation. You might hear
someone argue that industrial food is the American way because it's the
product of big business, which is the secret to our success as a nation. Today,
many Americans believe that the corporate sector should be as large and
powerful as possible, because this is the way to create the highest standard
of living for the greatest number of people. They believe that large corporations are necessary to provide the jobs, products, and economic prosperity
that make America great.

   This message has become part of the mantra that we live by. But it's only
a half-truth. According to University of California economist Kathryn Kobe,
as recently as 2002, small business accounted for as much as 48 percent of
the U.S. gross domestic product. This percentage has been in decline since
the beginning of the twenty-first century and especially since the recession

How Do You Maintain an Egalitarian Ideal in an Unequal Society?

The typical dictionary definition of
the American Dream is an ideal of
social equality that promises material abundance for all. To call it an
"ideal" is an elegant way of saying
it's how we think things *should*
be, not necessarily how they are.
But humans tend to interpret their
realities in such a way as to make it
appear that their ideals *are* reality.
So if we assume that the American
Dream is already fully realized, how
then does a person explain poverty? Often, they do it by placing
the blame on the poor themselves:
"If anyone is poor in America it's
because they're lazy." The handy
thing about this logical sleight of
hand is that you never have to
acknowledge inequality within the
system, so you never have to do
anything to fix it.

of 2009, after which, according to Kobe's 2012 report to the Small Business Administration, corporate profits recovered more quickly than those outside the corporate sector, reducing the share of the GDP produced by small businesses.

The Rest of the World Should Just Learn to Act Like Us. The Western lifestyle, meaning the one predominantly lived by Americans, is rapidly sweeping the globe—to the point where, in many social science textbooks, the word "globalization" is used interchangeably with "Westernization." Many of us Westerners think that's as it should be, since we believe that we have the highest standard of living in the world. Materially speaking, that's true. If a standard of living is measured by consumption, nobody makes, uses, and throws away as much stuff per capita as Americans.

But there's a problem with this assertion. According to National Geographic's Human Footprint project, if every human being alive today consumed Earth's resources at the rate of the average American, we'd need the equivalent of four Earths to keep up with the demand. It might very well be *impossible* for seven billion humans, and counting, to live like Westerners.

The Arguments You'll Hear

In many ways, local-sustainable living really does run contrary to most Americans' accepted view of the world. This may explain why some people—not most, not many, but *some*—may respond to the idea of eating locally as though doing this is a threat to them, because, in a sense, it is. It's a direct challenge to their worldview. Naturally, they may feel compelled to fight back, to defend their way of life. That's understandable. It also explains why your newfound food life may occasionally be greeted with insults, labels, name-calling, straw man arguments, and ad hominem attacks. Here are a few of the things people might say to you:

You Want Us All to Live in Poverty. Many people who come up against the unsustainability of American consumption draw this conclusion. Lower consumption means I have to live like a Spartan, do without, suffer. No, thanks!

Advocates of a low-impact lifestyle often get negative blowback from people who assume that the only choices are between keeping the status quo and vowing to live in grinding poverty. But this assumption misses the essential reason why many people criticize the Western level of consumption: that it's unsustainable in the long run because it damages and depletes the natural world.

Isn't there a third choice here? We're acknowledging that current Western levels of consumption are likely to prove to be unsustainable in the long run, but I've never heard anyone say this means we all need to live like the poor. What we're advocating is a move toward new modes of consumption that sustainably meet the needs of all people. It's not a choice between spreading it too thin or denying it to others. It's about a creative, diverse, all-ideas-on-the-table search for a *new* way to produce an abundant life for *everyone*.

You'd Rather Let People Starve Than Let Them Eat GMOs. A small minority of the folks within high-tech industries is quick to condemn anyone who suggests that maybe we shouldn't deploy a high-tech solution where a low-tech one works just as well. I've had students in my class who have taken this position, and now and again I've bumped into people who seem eager to make a straw man out of the viewpoint that urges caution when it comes to new technical innovations.

I've never met anyone who is patently anti-technology, but I have met quite a few people, myself included, who believe that new inventions require careful consideration. Any new technology comes with unintended consequences and costs, both overt ones and less obvious ones, and its full impact may not manifest until decades after the invention is deployed. These costs may be economic, environmental, or social. What may seem like a boon in the short run could cause worse problems in the long run. This, in a nutshell, is the reason why many people raise concerns over GMOs.

Dr. Vandana Shiva, in an article titled "The Golden Rice Hoax," makes precisely this argument against golden rice—the genetically engineered, vitamin A-rich superfood developed by Ingo Potrykus of the Swiss Federal Institute of Technology and Peter Beyer of the University of Freiberg. Shiva claims that golden rice is not the best solution to regional vitamin A deficiencies because the women of Bengal have historically grown more than a hundred varieties of semi-wild greens that can provide all the vitamin A the population needs, so long as they have access to the local resources it takes to grow them. She advocates that communities should cultivate local crops of these native plants, instead of an expensive, exclusive product that would amount to a handout. Her argument is not against technology, but *for* the self-sufficiency of her people.

Nobody Wants to Go Back to Digging Dirt and Kitchen Drudgery. People often react negatively to the suggestion that we could grow and cook more of our own food. They argue that they don't have time for it, which is their way of saying that they give these activities a low priority. There are plenty of other things that they *do* find the time for.

In spite of modern technological breakthroughs that have made farming and cooking easier, it's likely that doing these things will indeed result in a few more hours spent moving around outdoors and a little more time spent in the kitchen with loved ones. But we're not going back to the way things were. We're going forward.

We have new techniques and technologies that make growing and cooking food easier than it has ever been. We have new attitudes about gender roles and child rearing that will make it easier for family meals to become shared tasks. It will take some time and effort, but not as much as it did in the past, and it will not be as inequitably assigned as it was just a few decades ago. A move to local food is not a return to backbreaking farm labor and kitchen drudgery, but a first step toward a new way of life.

Sustainable Agriculture Is All Hype and Bad Science. I've read a few articles that claim pastured cattle would actually cause more damage to the environment than CAFO cattle, because pasture would need to be found for them and they would use more water because they walk around more. I'm just curious, on what data is this argument based?

You could argue that, at the moment, the ultimate sustainability of any agricultural method can't be verified, because we don't yet have the kind of megadata that it would take to accurately answer the kinds of "big picture" questions we're asking now—questions such as, what exactly will humankind's contribution of greenhouse gases do to the atmosphere? Precisely how much fossil fuel consumption is sustainable? How many people *can* Earth support?

As I wrote this book, I saw an opportunity to raise a slightly different set of questions. I think that if we reword the questions a bit, we'll be able to find more reliable answers. A question such as "Is organic milk really healthier?" is going to get a misleading answer because it begs another question, "Healthier than what?" And another, "What aspects of health are you comparing?" And especially, "What do you mean by *organic*?" We have to have realistic information about what these terms really mean, and about *all* the options, not just the ones that are currently popular.

The Names They May Call You

L abeling is a popular tactic among people who feel threatened. We've all done it. If we can stick a label on someone, they're a known quantity: "She's just one of *those*, and I've dealt with *them* before." Labeling is a form of judging, and judging is the antithesis of understanding. When I call someone by a label, I've stopped listening to him. Here are a few of the choice labels that people have tried to pin on me for living, thinking, and teaching the way that I do. As you adopt a new attitude toward food, some of these words may soon be headed your way:

Anti-God, Anti-American, Anti-Capitalist. If I find wisdom in any faith other than Christianity, or in a faith-free philosophy such as secular humanism, I must be anti-Christian. If I teach people what the natural sciences say about the evolution of life on this planet, I am anti-God. If I teach about the human suffering caused by the Trail of Tears, I must be anti-American. If I think that the urge to maximize profit has gone into overdrive, that big business has become too powerful, and that the marketplace does indeed need a certain amount of regulation in order to keep it from exploiting people or destroying the environment, I must be anti-capitalist.

Any time you suggest that views other than the prevailing one might be worthy of consideration, a small number of people will go on the warpath. To them, there's no room for a balanced point of view, no quarter for relativity.

How to respond? I've struggled with this question a lot. The people I admire most tend to respond to spates of name-calling by giving the labelers an opportunity to express themselves. They actually solicit the other person's opinion, and then they listen, carefully and sincerely, without arguing back. Sometimes, by doing this, they can at least lay a foundation for mutual respect.

Bleeding-Heart Liberal, Socialist. These words sound political to me, which is why I find them mind-blowing. I have no idea where I fall on the political spectrum, and I really don't care. I don't make my decisions based on what a particular political party advocates. I try to think about each issue independently. The ideal I'm striving for is to understand as many points of view as I can. I'm always on the lookout for ideas that could produce a happier, more equitable, and secure way of life for people. I'll consider any idea that claims it can do that. Does *that* point of view have a name? If so, call me one of those.

Greenie, Environmentalist. How did these terms ever get to be pejoratives? An environmentalist is someone who is working to assure that the natural world is not harmed or depleted. "Greenie" is a slang term for an environmentalist. Calling someone a negative name gives the caller a spike of adrenalized power, just as it did back in school days to call the large-framed girl "fatty" or the gentle guy who likes theater a "fag." I just can't figure out what's supposed to be negative about being plus-sized, theatrically inclined, or environmentally concerned.

Foodie, Food Snob. Local food advocates are sometimes called "foodies" for the same reasons environmentalists get called "greenies." A food snob, near as I can figure, is a term for anyone who turns up their noses at any dish that doesn't qualify as gourmet. This is the polar opposite of what most local food advocates really stand for, which is good, simple food available to all.

Many of us *are* crazy about great food. Some of us go into raptures at trying any kind of new cuisine, and a lot of us, because we love the stuff so much, have a passion for excellent food that's prepared with a creative flair. But I have just as much zeal for a simple baked potato. A snob is an elitist. Food snobbery is about using what you eat to place yourself in a category above other people. Local food does the opposite. It equalizes all people by rallying them around the common pleasure of eating.

Luddite. The first time somebody called me one of these, I had to look it up. This was the name given to English textile workers in the early nineteenth century who rebelled against the new weaving machines that threatened to destroy their livelihood. Folklore has it that these rebels organized around a young stockingmaker named Ned Ludd who smashed the equipment that was making him redundant. Today, the term is used to label someone who the labeler wants to dismiss as anti-industry, anti-automation, or anti-technology. As a hard-core devotee of indoor plumbing, this is definitely *not* me. I mean, *c'mon*—can't we just have a dialogue about solving the problems in a particular technology, without people trying to say we're utterly against it?

Hypocrite. A hypocrite is someone who doesn't practice what she preaches. If I appear this way to you, I won't say you're wrong. I'll say that I don't mean to be, that I'm sincerely trying to find a positive way to live and want to share what I find along the way. I'd suggest that if you see me acting in a way that seems hypocritical, you may not fully understand my point of view, especially because I haven't totally *arrived* as a local eater—I'm still learning and experimenting myself—and that I'm not a purist about very much at all. I'm a big believer in the idea of everything in moderation. As a student of human life, I think almost everything is negotiable. Except my morning coffee.

The English word "hypocrite" comes from the Greek *hypokrites*, or actor, and means "a person whose actions contradict stated belief."

If a hypocrite is one whose actions sometimes appear to contradict her beliefs, then we are all hypocrites. A conscious, informed opinion is a work in progress. It's always being tested and updated. The individual who holds it is always working to bring her actions in line with her beliefs. The task is never complete. If someone floats this word your way, you can wear it proudly, as a learning, growing creature who's not afraid to acknowledge her own messy contradictions.

Besides, if my actions *never* contradict my views, it might just be a sign that I'm adhering to my beliefs a little too rigidly. I've decided that it's okay to break my own rules once in a while, so long as I'm following them the majority of the time. In fact, I've come to a point where I sometimes break my own rules deliberately, just to see if they're still worth following.

No More Lunchbox Evangelism

In one of Charles Schulz's *Peanuts* comic strips, Lucy explains that she convinced a little boy at school that her religion was better than his. When asked how she did this, she replied, "I hit him with my lunchbox." This kind of argument has become a favorite debate tactic in the United States, especially when it comes to our impact on the environment.

Maybe we need to quit doing this.

We've just discussed some of the mind-sets that may predispose people to want to whack you with their metaphorical lunchboxes. When it happens, should you whip out your own lunchbox and fight back? Tempting as it is, it just seems as though there's enough of this already. Could we, just this once, create a national talking point that's a safe harbor for ideas instead of a battleground?

Lately, I've been meeting up with people from various walks of life who have impressed the heck out of me because of the way they respond to individuals whose viewpoints are different from theirs. They don't criticize,

Local Food: Your Best Hedge Against the Zombie Apocalypse

When the zombie apocalypse hits and the slavering undead are scrabbling at your door, *then* you'll be glad you opted into local food. A local food lifestyle leads you to keeping more food on hand—in your downstairs freezer, in your cabinets, in your fridge, and in your barbed-wire-enclosed backyard garden, which will prove vital in the event of a global attack of the re-animated. Your family won't have to wander decimated city streets in search of the last morsels. You can stay safe within your well-fortified, zombie-proof compound. Best of all, you won't have to resort to eating each other. (NOTE: This sidebar is lovingly dedicated, from my underground concrete bunker, to the folks who react to my interest in local food by labeling me a "survivalist.")

belittle, or try to prove how right they are. Instead, they do something extraordinary.

They listen to them.

These people's egos are not wrapped up in their opinions. They accept that individuals are going to have different points of view, and they try to learn as much as they can from every viewpoint they encounter. They examine as much data as they can, and they form their opinions based on a careful, thoughtful, ongoing examination of it. They are always ready to revise their perspective as new information becomes available. They seek out viewpoints that are different from theirs because they believe that solutions lie precisely in the place where individuals differ the most.

I want to be more like these people. And I really, *really* think that those of us who are talking about the American food system could benefit a lot from this attitude. This issue is so complex, and so important, that it would help to come at it with an all-ideas-on-the-table approach.

May Your Bliss Be Your Argument

English composition teachers claim that everything's an argument. By "argument," they don't mean "quarrel," but "point of view." In every action, we're communicating something about where we stand. This includes every decision we make about buying and consuming food.

This chapter has focused on the kinds of arguments that are made with words. But maybe the best way to convince people of the merits of an idea is not to say anything at all, but to simply live it. In the end, it might be the *outcome* of your choices that makes the greatest impression.

If eating locally brings you better health, warmer connections, and a deeper relationship with nature, the benefits of that choice will be obvious to the people you meet. They'll be making their own choices, and following their own paths, which will lead them to you. They'll be drawn to your light.

Poached Pears

After we realized that our autumn CSA bag was going to come stuffed with pears for the next few months, we started experimenting with pear recipes. This recipe makes a simple, healthy harvest-time dessert for a family of four.

4 large pears

1 cup honey

1/2 cup melted butter

1/2 cup water

4 cardamom pods

1 teaspoon cinnamon

1/4 teaspoon nutmeg

pinch of ginger

Place the pears in a small baking dish. Combine all other ingredients in a small saucepan and heat for five minutes, but don't boil. Pour the mixture over the pears. Bake pears at 325 degrees for about 30 minutes.

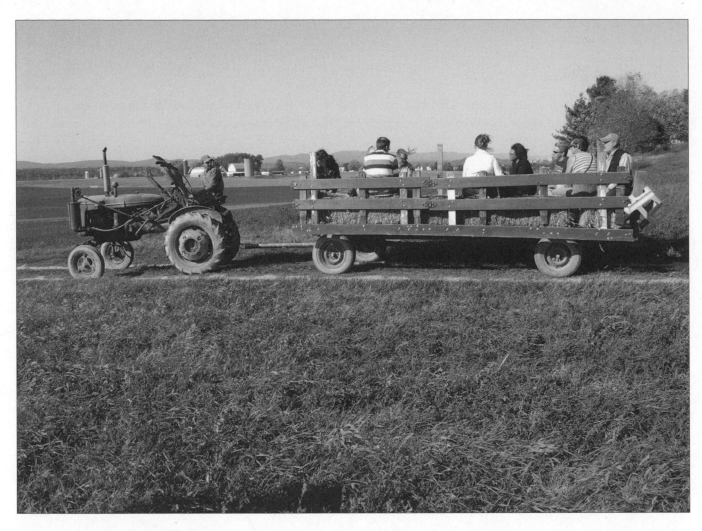

Visitors tour Nick Maravell's farm by tractor.

Last Thoughts

Local Food in a Global Future

To be a sailor of the world, bound for all ports. —*Walt Whitman*

Thank you for coming all the way to the end of the book with me. We've defined local food and discussed where to find it, how to afford it, prepare it, and make room for it in a busy lifestyle. We've talked about the ways a homegrown food economy can build families and communities, safeguard its environment, and promote a more equitable world. There's really only one thing left to do: let's see where it will take us in the future.

At the end of last semester, one of my noncredit students, most of whom are over fifty-five, sent me a thank-you note in which she wrote, "I'd grown so despairing of the future that it had made me glad I'm old and won't be here much longer. You've given me the first positive outlook I've had in a long time."

She's not the only one who thinks we're facing a bleak future. Numerous experts from diverse scientific backgrounds point to a moment of reckoning looming on the horizon, an era of environmental and economic tipping points, in which our current way of life could cease to be viable and we'll be forced to adopt a new way. They can show some pretty compelling evidence. They could be wrong. But in case they prove to be right, it might be prudent to start taking steps to prepare for this scenario.

We've already arrived at a point where we need to start making decisions as a global community. Our atmosphere and oceans, among other resources, have been described as a global commons. It may prove to be impossible to manage the use of these things, to avoid damage and overexploitation, unless all nations cooperate with a plan to protect them.

If this is the case, we no longer have the luxury of thinking about each other as "us" versus "them," as tribe against tribe, or nation against nation. It may now be imperative for us to think, plan, and act as one community. After so many millennia of practicing racism, sexism, classism, nationalism, and ethnocentrism, this might prove to be a tall order.

If we want to work together, we'll need to focus on what unites us, rather than what divides us.

In some of my noncredit classes, I do a little thought experiment. It goes like this: a knock comes at your door and you open it to find a little green alien standing there, holding a clipboard. He says, "Excuse me, I'm writing the definitive book about human beings. Can you give me the inside scoop on what it's like to be human?"

I ask the students to give me all the words that they believe best describe our kind. In every class in which I've done this experiment, the one word that always makes the list is greed. Usually, this one comes up long before creativity, curiosity, or compassion.

Greed. Really?

I know that many religious traditions have a lot to say about greed. It's viewed as a sin, as a severance of the relationship between us and the divine. I get this. It makes sense to me. But some of the voices that have entered the dialogue about the nature of human existence frame greed not so much as a sin but as a mistake. It's assuming that to meet the needs of the self, we must put the self before others. Yet, to do that is to misunderstand the nature of the human self and what it *really* needs.

We are social animals. We can't survive without fellow humans. We can't thrive without belonging to a group. For all creatures like us, the best way to serve self is not to focus on self-interest but to focus on serving loved ones, family, community. Serving each other in a loving bond is not just a nice sentiment. It's also a human need, right alongside air, water, food, and shelter. And for this reason, any design we create for our future needs to have community at its heart.

One of the things I love most about anthropology is that it can give you the hard-core scientific evidence to back up the notion of human equality. Any anthropologist can provide you with loads of evidence to show that, among living human beings, there's no such thing as "race." All humans alive today share 99.5 percent or more of our genes in common with all other living humans. That's way too much genetic similarity to leave room for races. The visual markers we use to distinguish race are based on nothing more than phenotypic differences, meanings we place on surface-level traits such as skin color. We're the same inside.

Similarly, there's no evidence to support the idea that upper class people are smarter, harder working, or morally superior to lower class people. Whenever social scientists have tried to justify classes with biological evidence, they end up doing bad science. They simply use the traits of their own group as the ultimate benchmark of the highest class.

Likewise, there's no scientifically valid evidence to support the idea that any nation is inherently superior to another. As the folks who have visited the International Space Station are always trying to tell us, national boundaries are arbitrary. We may like a trait of one nation better than another, but it's nonsensical to rank the traits of one nation according to the standards of another. The history of each nation is unique: a specific response to a specific set of circumstances. The principle of cultural relativism says that if you judge one nation to be inferior because of some perceived fault or flaw, you lose the ability to see faults and flaws within your own nation.

There isn't even evidence to support the idea that we're an inherently violent species. Sadly, historical records seem to indicate that the majority of human societies have resorted to collective violence occasionally, or often. But a small handful of societies haven't: for instance, the Semai of West Malaysia, the Hutterites of the United States and Canada, or the Ju/Wasi of Namibia. The fact that there are at least a few nonviolent societies makes the case that violent conflict is not a biological imperative.

What the data *does* support is the idea that we're all one species of highly social animal, and we adapt our way of life to the circumstances in which we find ourselves. So any given culture, and any given society, is no more and no less than a unique adaptation to its particular set of circumstances. When you view it that way, you realize that you can't judge one way of life as superior or inferior to any other.

But if all this is really the case, why is it so hard for people to recognize the fundamental equality of humankind?

This past semester, when I was explaining the idea of cultural relativism, one student said, "I disagree. I think there's something seriously wrong with the people of _____ (you can fill in the blank with whichever country is currently unpopular). How can you possibly say they're just as good as us? How can you excuse all those human rights violations?"

This student is assuming that the reason for these atrocities must be a result of something inherently flawed in *those* people. He's thinking, we're a better kind of creature than them, and we would never do such a thing.

Well, that's one way of looking at it.

Here's another: all humans are the same kind of being, all capable of the same things. When a society manifests violence and hatred, it's not because they are inferior human beings, because humans everywhere are fundamentally the same. It's that something in their environment is producing that response. Any one of us, placed within the same circumstances, might respond the same way. If we shift from denouncing the people to examining their circumstances, we see a way forward that doesn't lead us to hatred, judgment, and blame.

It's only when people are willing to step outside their own worldviews that they have any hope of seeing things from a different perspective.

I choose to believe human equality is an achievable goal, because I can see that the inequalities in the world are not biological but human-made. If there's one thing anthropology teaches about human beings, it's that we're adaptable. Anything within human society that is cultural, and therefore learned, is subject to change.

What if, in the near future, self-interest, group interest, and national interest transform into *global* interest, and "taking care of one's own" comes to mean an active concern and responsibility for all human beings, and all life systems?

According to certain forward-looking economists, within the next few decades, we may reach a tipping point in which the current post-industrial way of life, characterized by high consumption and commercial exchange, ceases to be viable. We're likely to see a future in which most jobs are lower paying than today's, and the average worker holds several jobs at once. By necessity, people will consume less. Economist Hugo Garcia, in a *Futurist* magazine article titled "Consumption 2.0," claimed that the trend in future decades will be toward less ownership of stuff, especially big-ticket items such as homes and cars.

Economist Marjorie Kelly, in her book *Owning Our Future: The Emerging Ownership Revolution*, envisions a future in which business owners and employees make abundant profits, but nobody gets rich at the expense of someone else. Worldwide, economic strength may no longer be conceived in terms of competition, but in terms of security and equality: all people in all communities enjoying sustainable abundance.

How does this picture relate to our discussion of local food? Because food is the lifeblood of any society. The system by which a group obtains its food influences its form of economic exchange, political organization, family structure, and social roles. Whereas before, we tended to think one-dimensionally about our eating habits, we're now learning to take a holistic view of food. We can see it as one part of a bigger picture. When enough of us change the way we eat, we set up a ripple effect of change throughout our society.

The future that we're rising to meet is going to make new demands on us. Once we're able to recognize our responsibility to fellow humans, we'll be ready to take the next step: to recognize our responsibility to other living things. We're the only creatures on this planet who know we're *on* a planet. Maybe that recognition comes with a responsibility. For the past several decades, we've earned a reputation for being planet killers. But we might also, possibly, choose to become planet healers.

I like thinking of us as the guardians of the planet, instead of the worst thing that ever happened to it.

As a budding futurist, I sometimes try to visualize humans of the future. Of course, as a card-carrying meliorist, I choose to assume the positive. Here's what I see:

As a whole, twenty-second century humans are happier, more playful, loving, and creative than we are today. They know far more about their world than most of us know about ours, and yet they experience a far deeper sense of mystery, awe, and wonder about all the things that they don't know. Their happiness comes, not from owning or acquiring, or even from achieving, but from serving other living things. They can appreciate art, poetry, and music far more deeply than we can, but they do not require these things for entertainment because they derive fascination and intense satisfaction from observing the world around them.

They are fiercely protective of their planet, all the forms of life on it, and all the complex interwoven webs that connect them. They do not hate, make war, or exploit. They experience differences between one another as adventures and learning opportunities.

These future humans are responsible, clear-minded, and far-seeing, yet spontaneous and full of wonder. They are quick to laugh and deeply affectionate. They feed anyone who is hungry, heal anyone who is sick or hurt, and take in anyone who is an outsider. They recognize a fundamental equality in all human beings. They treat each new person they meet as a friend.

They are like us on our best days.

According to many of the brightest minds of our day, change is in the wind, and we will live to see it. It may be less a question of whether it will happen, but whether it will be beneficial for humanity or disastrous. I've decided to assume that in the long run it will be good. It may complicate our children's lives for a time, but *their* children's lives will be richer for it. We may get blown about a bit, but when the dust settles, we're going to love what we see.

We're taking the first steps toward that future now, beginning with reclaiming our means of fulfilling the most basic need we have: the need for sustenance. By choosing to obtain our food from carefully considered sources, by eating with our eyes fully open, we are doing something good— and the effects of our choices will be felt for generations to come.

Sources and Recommended Reading

Ahmed, Nafeez. "Former BP Geologist: Peak Oil is Here and It Will 'Break Economies." *The Guardian,* Dec. 2013. Web. 21 Mar. 2014.

"American Dream." *Merriam-Webster.com.* Merriam-Webster, 2014. Web. 21 Mar. 2014.

An Inconvenient Truth. Dir. Davis Guggenheim. Perf. Al Gore, Billy West. Paramount, 2006. DVD.

Anderson, Chris. *FREE: The Future of a Radical Price.* New York: Hyperion. 2009. Print.

Andrews, James. "Imports and Exports: The Global Beef Trade." *Food Safety News,* 18 Nov. 2013. Web. 28 Mar. 2014.

Baker Creek Heirloom Seeds. *Good Seeds: 1500 Rare, Non-GMO Seeds, 2014 Catalog.* Mansfield MO: RareSeeds Publishing, LLC. 2014.

Beavan, Colin. *No Impact Man: Adventures of a Guilty Liberal Who Attempts to Save the Planet, and the Discoveries He Makes About Himself and Our Way of Life in the Process.* London: Picador. 2010. Print.

Bell, Janice F., Jeffrey S. Wilson, and Gilbert C. Liu. "Neighborhood Greenness and 2-Year Changes in Body Mass Index of Children and Youth." *American Journal of Preventive Medicine,* Vol. 35, Issue 6. Dec. 2008. Web. 23 Mar. 2014.

Ben-Ami, Daniel. "Why People Hate Fat Americans." *Spiked,* 9 Sept. 2005. Web. 23 Mar. 2014.

Benbrook, Charles, et al. "New Evidence Confirms the Nutritional Superiority of Plant-based Organic Foods." *PLoS ONE,* Dec. 2013. Web. 23 Mar. 2014.

"Big business." *Merriam-Webster.com.* Merriam-Webster, 2014. Web. 1 Apr. 2014.

Cable News Network (CNN.) "Are Humans Endangered if Cattle Dine on Chicken Manure?" CNN. 23 Aug. 1997. Web. 25 Mar. 2014.

Cable News Network (CNN.) "Feeding the Future: Saving Agricultural Biodiversity." CNN. 6 Sept. 2009. Web. 25 Mar. 2014.

Carsten, Janet E. "Cooking Money: Gender and the Symbolic Transformation of Means of Exchange in a Malay Fishing Village." *Money and the Morality of Exchange*, J. Parry and M. Block, eds. Cambridge, MA: Cambridge University Press. 1989. Print.

Cockrall-King, Jennifer. *Food and the City.* Amherst, NY: Prometheus Books. 2012. Print.

Collingham, Lizzie. *The Taste of War: World War II and the Battle for Food.* New York: Penguin. 2013. Print.

"Commodity." *Merriam-Webster.com.* Merriam-Webster, 2014. Web. 21 Mar. 2014.

Consumer Reports Magazine. "How Safe is That Chicken? Most Tested Broilers Were Contaminated." *Consumer Reports Magazine.* Jan. 2010. Web. 28 Mar. 2014.

Counts, David. "Too Many Bananas, Not Enough Pineapples, and No Watermelon At All: Three Object Lessons in Living with Reciprocity." *The Humbled Anthropologist: Tales from the Pacific,* Philip DeVita, ed. Belmont, CA: Wadsworth. 1990. Print.

Delind, Laura B. "Parma: The Story of Hog Hotels and Local Resistance." *Pigs, Profits, and Rural Communities.* Kendall Thu and E. Paul Durrenberger, eds. Albany, NY: University of California Press. 1998. Print.

Diamond, Jared. *Collapse: How Societies Choose to Fail or Succeed.* New York: Penguin. 2005. Print.

Diamond, Jared. *Guns, Germs, and Steel: The Fates of Human Societies.* New York: W. W. Norton & Company. 1999. Print.

Douglas, Mary. *Purity and Danger: An Analysis of Concepts of Pollution and Taboo.* New York: Routledge, New Ed edition. 1984. Print.

Ember, Carol R., Melvin Ember, and Peter N. Peregrine. *Anthropology, 12th edition.* Upper Saddle River, NJ: Pearson. 2010. Print.

Environmental Working Group. "Farm Subsidies in California: Skewed Priorities and Gross Inequities." Environmental Working Group. 1 May 2010. Web. 26 Mar. 2014.

Fed Up. Dir. Stephanie Soechtig. Perf. Michelle Simon. 2014. DVD.

Fiese, Barbara H., A. Hammons, D. Grigsby-Toussaint. "Family Mealtimes: A Contextual Approach to Understanding Childhood Obesity." *Economics and Human Biology.* 2012. Web. 23 Mar. 2014.

Fisher, Roger, and William Ury. *Getting to YES: Negotiating Agreement Without Giving In.* New York: Penguin. 1983. Print.

Food, Inc. Dir. Robert Kenner. Perf. Michael Pollan, Eric Schlosser. Magnolia Pictures. 2008. DVD.

Frederick County, Md., Division of Business Development and Retention. *Frederick Farm Guide 2012.* Print.

Garcia, Hugo. "Consumption 2.0." *Futurist,* Jan.-Feb. 2013. Print.

Genkinger, Jeanine, and Anita Koushik. "Meat Consumption and Cancer Risk." *PLoS Medicine,* Vol. 4(12) Dec. 2007. Web. 22 Mar. 2014.

Goleman, Daniel. *Ecological Intelligence: The Hidden Impacts of What We Buy.* New York: Crown Business. 2010. Print.

Goodall, Chris. *Sustainability: All That Matters.* Burr Ridge, IL: McGraw-Hill. 2013. Print.

Grandin, Temple. *Animals Make Us Human: Creating the Best Life for Animals.* Boston, MA: Houghton Mifflin Harcourt. 2008. Print.

Gustafson, Katherine. *Change Comes to Dinner: How Vertical Farmers, Urban Growers, and Other Innovators are Revolutionizing the Way America Eats.* London: St. Martin's Griffin. 2012. Print.

Harris, Marvin. *Cows, Pigs, Wars, and Witches: The Riddles of Culture.* New York: Vintage. 1974. Print.

Harvard School of Public Health. "Calcium and Milk: What's Best for Your Bones and Health?" Harvard School of Public Health. 2014. Web. 25 Mar. 2014.

Hewitt, Ben. *The Town that Food Saved: How One Community Found Vitality in Local Food.* Emmaus, PA: Rodale Books, Reprint edition. 2011. Print.

Hill, Adriene. "Which States Have the Most Farmers' Markets? Where's My Nearest Market?" Markeplace: Easy, Sustainable Answers. 4 Aug. 2010. Web. 24 Mar. 2014.

Hughes, Jonathan, and Louis P. Cain. *American Economic History, 5th Edition.* Reading, MA: Addison, Wesley, Longman. 1998. Print.

Huhn, Laura B., and William Halal. "Major Transformations to 2100: Highlights from the TechCast Project." *Futurist,* Sept.-Oct. 2012. Print.

Human Rights Watch. "Immigrant Workers in the United States Meat and Poultry Industry." Human Rights Watch. 15 Dec. 2005. Web. 10 Apr. 2014.

In Organics We Trust. Dir. Kip Pator. Perf. Nyeila Grissom, Linda Domeyer, Ben Skolnik. Pasture Pictures, 2012. DVD.

Kaiser Family Foundation. "Generation M2: Media in the Lives of 8-to-18-Year-Olds." Kaiser Family Foundation. Jan. 2010. Web. 27 Mar. 2014.

Kelley, Marjorie. *Owning Our Future: The Emerging Ownership Revolution.* San Francisco, CA: Berrett-Koehler. 2012. Print.

Kingsolver, Barbara. *Animal, Vegetable, Miracle: A Year of Food Life.* New York: Harper Perennial. 2007. Print.

Klare, Michael. *The Race for What's Left: The Global Scramble for the World's Last Resources.* London: Picador, Reprint edition. 2012. Print.

Kobe, Kathryn. "Small Business GDP: Update 2002-2010." *Small Business Administration*, Jan. 2012. Web. 22 Mar. 2014.

Kotler, Steve. *Abundance: The Future Is Better Than You Think.* New York: Free Press. 2012. Print.

Kottak, Conrad Phillip. *Window on Humanity: A Concise Introduction to Anthropology.* New York: McGraw-Hill. 2012. Print.

Krotz, Daniel. "Small Farms and the Farm Subsidy Scandal." *Huffington Post,* 3 Feb. 2011. Web. 26 Mar. 2014.

Kurlansky, Mark. *Salt: A World History.* New York: Penguin Books. 2003. Print.

Lappé, Frances Moore, and Joseph Collins. *Food First: Beyond the Myth of Scarcity.* Boston, MA: Houghton-Mifflin. 1977. Print.

Leakey, Richard. *The 6th Extinction: Patterns of Life and the Future of Humankind.* Sioux City, IA: Anchor, Reprint edition. 1996. Print.

Lee, James H. "Hard at Work in a Jobless Future." *Futurist,* Mar.-Apr. 2012. Print.

Lee, Richard Borshay. "Eating Christmas in the Kalahari." *Annual Editions: Anthropology 10/11*, 33. Elvio Angeloni, ed. Dubuque, Iowa: McGraw-Hill. 2009. Print.

Li, Sophia. "Stressed Aquifers Around the Globe." *New York Times* Green blog. Web. 13 Aug. 2013.

Liittschwager, David. *A World in One Cubic Foot: Portraits of Biodiversity.* Chicago: University of Chicago Press. 2012. Print.

Lin, Meihwa. *The Learning Annex Presents Feng Shui: The Smarter Approach to the Ancient Art of Feng Shui.* New York: Wiley. 2004. Print.

Louv, Richard. *The Nature Principle: Reconnecting With Life in a Virtual Age.* Chapel Hill, NC: Algonquin Books, Reprint edition. 2012. Print.

McMillan, Tracie. "Where Does Your Grocery Money Go? Mostly Not to the Farmers." Cable News Network. 8 Aug. 2012. Web. 27 Mar. 2014.

"Meliorism." *Merriam-Webster.com.* Merriam-Webster, 2014. Web. 21 Mar. 2014.

Mintz, Sydney. *Sweetness and Power: The Place of Sugar in Modern History.* New York: Penguin. 1985. Print.

Moss, Michael. *Salt, Sugar, Fat: How the Giants Hooked Us.* New York: Random House. 2013. Print.

National Geographic: Human Footprint. Dir. Clive Maltby. Perf. Elizabeth Vargas. Touch Productions. 2008. DVD.

Nelson, Richard. "Understanding Eskimo Science: Traditional Hunters' Insights into the Natural World are Worth Rediscovering." *Audubon*, Sept.-Oct. 1993. Print.

Owings, Lisa. *Sustainable Agriculture (Innovative Technologies).* Minneapolis, MN: Abdo Publishing Company. 2013. Print.

Oz, Mehmet. "What to Eat Now: The Anti-Food-Snob Diet." *Time Magazine,* 3 Dec. 2012. Print.

Paxson, Heather. "Locating Value in Artisanal Cheese: Reverse Engineering *Terroir* for New Landscapes." *American Anthropologist*, Vol. 112(3) 2010. Print.

Park, Michael Alan. *Introducing Anthropology: An Integrated Approach, 5th Edition.* New York: McGraw-Hill. 2011. Print.

Petrini, Carlo. *The Slow Food Revolution: A New Culture for Eating and Living.* New York: Rizzoli. 2006. Print.

Physicians Committee for Responsible Medicine. "Health Concerns About Dairy Products." Physicians Committee for Responsible Medicine, n.d. Web. 25 Mar. 2014.

Physicians Committee for Responsible Medicine. "Meat Consumption and Cancer Risk." Physicians Committee for Responsible Medicine, n.d. Web. 22 Mar. 2014.

Physicians Committee for Responsible Medicine. "USDA's New MyPlate Icon At Odds With Federal Subsidies for Meat, Dairy." Physicians Committee for Responsible Medicine. 2 June 2011. Web. 27 Mar. 2014.

Pinker, Steven. *The Better Angels of Our Nature: Why Violence Has Declined.* New York: Viking Adult. 2010. Print.

Pollan, Michael. *Food Rules: An Eater's Manual.* New York: Penguin. 2009. Print.

Pollan, Michael. *In Defense of Food: An Eater's Manifesto.* New York: Penguin. 2008. Print.

Pollan, Michael. *The Omnivore's Dilemma: A Natural History of Four Meals.* New York: Penguin. 2006. Print.

Putnam, Robert. *Bowling Alone: The Collapse and Revival of American Community.* New York: Simon & Schuster. 2000. Print.

Rainforest Alliance. "Banana." Rainforest Alliance, n.d. Web. 25 Mar. 2014.

Robbins, John. *The Food Revolution: How Your Diet Can Help Save Your Life and Our World.* San Francisco, CA: Conari Press. 2001. Print.

Robarchek, Clayton. "Motivations and Material Causes: On the Explanation of Conflict and War." *The Anthropology of War.* Jonathan Hass, ed. New York: Cambridge University Press. 1990. Print.

Robbins, Richard H. *Cultural ANTHRO.* Belmont, CA: Wadsworth. 2012. Print.

Rosset, Peter M. *The Multiple Functions and Benefits of Small Farm Agriculture in the Context of Global Trade Negotiations.* Institute for Food and Development Policy Brief, 4. Sept. 1999. Web. 29 Mar. 2014.

Rowney, Kim. *Growing Vegetables: Vegetables for All Seasons.* New York: Metro Books. 2004. Print.

Ruppenthal, R.J. *Fresh Food From Small Spaces: The Square-Inch Gardener's Guide to Year-Round Growing, Fermenting, and Sprouting.* White River Junction, VT: Chelsea Green. 2008. Print.

Salatin, Joel. *Folks, This Ain't Normal: A Farmer's Advice for Happier Hens, Healthier People, and a Better World.* New York: Center Street, Reprint edition. 2012. Print.

Salatin, Joel. *The Sheer Ecstasy of Being a Lunatic Farmer.* Swoope, VA: Polyface. 2010. Print.

Schlosser, Eric. *Fast Food Nation: The Dark Side of the All-American Meal.* Boston, MA: Mariner. 2012. Print.

Schonwald, Josh. *The Taste of Tomorrow: Dispatches from the Future of Food.* New York: Harper. 2012. Print.

Schulz, Charles. "Peanuts." 8 Dec. 1980. United Features Syndicate.

Schwartz, Barry. *The Paradox of Choice: Why More Is Less.* New York: HarperCollins. 2005. Print.

Shein, Christopher. *The Vegetable Gardener's Guide to Permaculture: Creating an Edible Ecosystem.* Portland, OR: Timber Press. 2013. Print.

Shiva, Vandana. "The Golden Rice Hoax: When Public Relations Replaces Science." San Francisco State University, n.d. Web. 22 Mar. 2014.

Shuman, Michael. *The Small Mart Revolution: How Local Businesses Are Beating the Global Competition.* San Francisco, CA: Berrett-Koehler. 2007. Print.

Slama, Jim. "Will Feds Bankrupt Small Farms With Safety Rules?" *Huffington Post,* 7 Nov. 2013. Web. 21 Jan. 2014.

Smith, Lawrence. *The World in 2050: Four Forces Shaping Civilization's Northern Future.* New York: Plume, Reprint edition. 2011. Print.

Strathern, Andrew. *The Rope of Moka: Big Men and Ceremonial Exchange in Mount Hagen, New Guinea.* London: Cambridge University Press, 1977. Print.

Supersize Me. Dir. Morgan Spurlock. Perf. Morgan Spurlock, Daryl Isaacs, Chemeeka Walker. The Con, 2004. DVD.

Unitarian Universalist Association. "Our Beliefs and Principles." *Unitarian Universalist Association,* n.d. Web. 23 Mar. 2014.

United States Department of Agriculture. "Organic Milk." USDA Agricultural Marketing Service. 28 May 2010. Web. 24 Mar. 2014.

WebMD. "The Truth About Sugar Addiction." WebMD 2014. Web. 26 Mar. 2014.

Wiggington, Eliot, and students. *The Foxfire Books*. Sioux City, IA: Anchor. 1977. Print.

Wolman, David. *The End of Money: Counterfeiters, Preachers, Techies, Dreamers—and the Coming Cashless Society*. Cambridge, MA: Da Capo Press. 2013. Print.

World Health Organization and UNICEF. "Progress on Drinking Water and Sanitation: 2012 Update." 2012. Web. 27 Mar. 2014.

Zehner, Ozzie. *Green Illusions: The Dirty Secrets of Clean Energy and the Future of Environmentalism*. Lincoln, NE: University of Nebraska Press. 2012. Print.

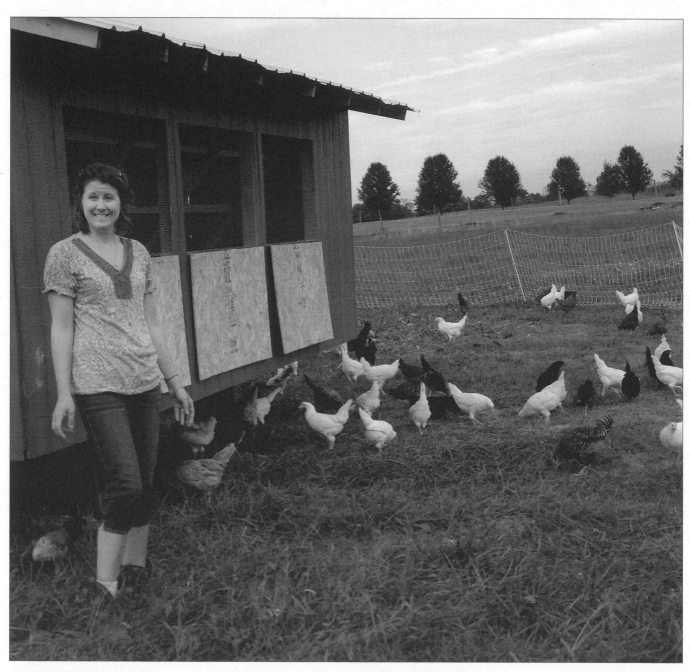

Abby Brusco of Local Harvest is pastured with a few chickens (see page 119).

Resources

Finding and Buying Local Food

Coop Directory Service: *www.coopdirectory.org*

Field to Plate: *www.fieldtoplate.com*

LocalHarvest, Inc.: *www.localharvest.com*

Monterey Bay Aquarium Seafood Watch: *www.seafoodwatch.org*

National Agricultural Statistics Service: *www.nass.usda.gov*

USDA Farmers' Market Search: *http://search.ams.usda.gov/farmersmarkets*

Organizations That Support Local, Sustainable, and Equitable Food

Fairtrade International: *www.fairtrade.net*

Food and Agriculture Organization of the United Nations: *www.fao.org*

Food Co-op Initiative: *www.foodcoopinitiative.coop*

The Food Project: *www.thefoodproject.org*

Humane Farm Animal Care: *www.certifiedhumane.org*

Humanitarian Aid Groups Devoted to Food Self-Sufficiency

Farm Aid: *www.farmaid.org*

Feeding America: *www.feedingamerica.org*

Heifer International: *www.heifer.org*

Oxfam America: *www.oxfamamerica.org*

Oxfam International: *www.oxfam.org*

Save the Children: *www.savethechildren.org*

United Nations Children's Fund: *www.unicef.org*

WaterAid America: *www.wateraid.org*

World Neighbors: *www.wn.org*

Support for Home Gardeners

American Community Gardening Association: *www.communitygarden.org*

Backyard Beekeepers Association: *www.beeculture.com.*

Permaculture Farming Blog: *www.permaculturefarming.org*

National Gardening Association: *www.garden.org*

United States National Arboretum Gardening Page: *www.usna.usda.gov/Gardens/gardeningr.html*

Acknowledgments

My sincerest thanks go to Daniel Kohan of Ruka Press for helping me take this book from wishful thinking to reality. Rapturous gratitude goes to my husband, Al Castillo, for fearless proofreading, tireless fact-checking, and boundless inspiration. I'd also like to express my deepest appreciation to Mary Kathryn and Andrew Barnet of Open Book Farm, Zoe Brittain and Sally Fulmer of the Common Market, Tony Brusco of Hometown Harvest, Molly C. Haviland of the Living Soil Compost Lab, Dr. Elaine Ingham of Soil Foodweb, Megan Lanasa of The Breadery, Nick Maravell of Nick's Organic Farm, Kathy MacFarland of Baker Creek Seed Company, Lois Pruitt of Bailey's Gems, Melissa Schulte of Black Ankle Vineyards, J'aime and Christian Sparrow of the Sunbird Food Truck, Stacy of Stacy's Tortillas, family physician Dr. Louise Steirmorowski, Jeff Taylor of Tuscarora Organic Growers, Christine Van Bloem of The Kitchen Studio, and certified arborist J. D. Willoughby for their guidance and contributions to this book. Many, many thanks to all of you. I'm in awe of your wisdom and expertise!

Index

Eat Local for Less Events and Classes

For information on upcoming classes and events, please visit:

www.eatlocalforlessbook.com

Follow Julie Castillo on Twitter:

@CastilloJulie

@EatLocalforLess

Cerulean Blues
A Personal Search for a Vanishing Songbird
by Katie Fallon

"Birds have the power to captivate, even change lives. Told here is the story of a woman who could and a small, blue, bellwether bird that increasingly cannot maintain itself in this world of our making. *Cerulean Blues* is part journey, part documentary, and wholly engaging; a tribute to a bird that bridges continents with its wings and to a rising star among contemporary nature writers."
—*Pete Dunne, Cape May Bird Observatory*

Among the Ancients
Adventures in the Eastern Old Growth Forests
by Joan Maloof

"An ode to lost old-growth forests everywhere, and a celebration of those few that remain. Joan Maloof simultaneously writes with the precision of a scientist and the passion of a poet. *Among the Ancients* will have you looking at all forests—young and old—with a new eye."   —*Gary K. Meffe, co-author,* Principles of Conservation Biology

Horseshoe Crab
Biography of a Survivor
by Anthony D. Fredericks

"In this entertaining tribute to 445-million years of horseshoe crabs, Fredericks challenges readers near and far from coastal beaches to embrace the conservation of these important creatures."
—*Booklist*

The Pipeline and the Paradigm
Keystone XL, Tar Sands, and the Battle to Defuse the Carbon Bomb
by Samuel Avery

"Sometimes a book comes along that captures a historical moment and records it in the making. This is such a book. If you want to know why this could be the battle that defines our generation, read it, then get involved and join history."
—*Paul Gilding, author of* The Great Disruption

"His finely researched book blazes with hope."
—*Publisher's Weekly*

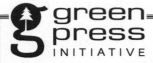